Live Longer and Healthier Now!

The ultimate guide to physical, emotional and financial health

by EVAN L. LIPKIS MD

To order additional copies of this book, contact:
Evan L. Lipkis MD
1-866-775-7628
www.DrLipkis.com
17025-LIPK

CONTENTS

Foreword

Live Longer and Healthier Now! is designed to give you the latest and most practical information about your health. It is a work that I will update regularly because the health field is constantly changing.

I will help you to slice through the controversies in medicine. This is a manual for life. Why, it's like having a doctor in your house! I'm not just going to tell you about weight loss, headaches, cancer prevention and cholesterol. I also will inform you about parenting, drugs, marriage, vitamins, alternative strategies and even outstanding investment ideas. This is a guide for life that you can't be without.

How can I write about such a broad range of information, you ask? Actually the answer is quite simple. I love to read and I'm enthusiastic about life. Additionally, I've made and seen so many mistakes that I'm your life's guru.

No doubt, I'm forever a student of life and always learning. In this valuable guide, I have distilled the best "pearls of wisdom" so that you will ultimately become healthier and wealthier. **Sure, always consult your doctor, lawyer and accountant before proceeding with my practical pointers.** These valuable professionals should always be a part of your team.

Finally, an excellent complement to this handbook is my free *Health and Wealth Newsletter*. Go to **www.DrLipkis.com** and click on the button that says "free newsletter." Enter your e-mail address and I will continue to keep you up-to-date with regard to standard and alternative medical strategies. At this site you can visit our archives of all the past valuable newsletters. The website also contains a superb vitamin store.

If you have a healthy mind and body, you're always in the ball game. Even if you make mistakes, you can always get back up on your feet. Armed with the power of this book, your life should go into extra innings!

"Live long, laugh often and love much."

Evan L. Lipkis, M.D.

Dedication

I dedicate this book to my wife, Dr. Sheree Lipkis, who always believed in my creative concepts. Without her support, I would never have had the home environment to be able to accomplish this work.

My daughter Aimee has been an inspiration to me. She has challenged me on so many subjects and has broadened my horizons.

I can't even begin to express the deep love that I have for these two outstanding people.

My office staff at Advanced Center for Total Health Care has helped me to build a great practice. I would never be the internist I am today without them. They are Judy Lieberman, Sheila Mozin, Julia Kaminski, Margaret Burgraff, Marilyn Keippel, Melissa Keippel, Michelle Brown, Cheryl Shapiro, Catherine Amoroso, Kathryn Kellen, Linda Wagner, Frances Rosendorn, Carolyn Rubel, Mona Schmidt, Sandy Shapero, Lauren Kornick, Kristal Jennings, Apeksha Shah and Georgia Dalakouras. Many thanks to my associates: Dr. Susan Shapiro, Dr. David Sommerfeld, Donna Wittert, N.P., Jan Kasner, C.P.T., Linda Clinton, R.D., Lynn Freedman, R.D., Michail Pys, L.M.T., and Judy Hild, M.A.

I am grateful for the guidance of my attorneys, Ira Leavitt, Gene Slade and Ted Shapero. My accountant, Steve Isenstein, always keeps my business on track.

I appreciate the strong educational upbringing that my parents, Harriet and Bernie Lipkis, provided me. I also appreciate the support of my sister, Lila George.

I am thankful for the support of my mother-in-law, Sylvia Balkin, my brother-in-law, Barry Balkin and my sister-in-law, Linda Balkin. My cousins Dorothy Ossoff and Sue Rogull have always supported my ideas. Their steadfast belief in me is greatly appreciated.

I am grateful to the many friends who inspired me to write this book, including Judy Katz, Paul Katz, Marcie Nach, Ralph Nach, Tami Slade, Gene Slade and Doug Cummings. I also appreciate the support of Jim Graziano, my marketing guru, and Connie Pagano, my hairstylist for more than four decades.

Many thanks to the staff at the Abington of Glenview, a superb nursing facility.

I appreciate the constructive feedback from Dr. Chris Leman, who also developed the title for this book. I am also grateful to Linda Youngman for her careful editing.

I also dedicate this book to the memory of seven thoughtful family members and friends who always believed in me; my father-in-law, Israel Balkin, Dr. Derek Miller, Paul Kerstein, Bert Warsaw, Terry Appell-Greenblatt, Irv Price and Harry Ossoff. Their guidance and kindness will never be forgotten.

Finally, my patients have been an inspiration to me. Their intelligent questions have been the driving force behind this book. Thank you for your loyalty and support.

Chapter One

Common Conditions

Here is a list of common conditions that I as an internist see almost every day in my office. Millions of people worldwide have these problems. Here is the latest information to help you get better!

Alcoholism

This disease is both genetic and behavioral. If you have at least 2 "yes" answers to the following questions, there is a good chance that you have alcoholism: Have you tried to cut down your drinking? Are you annoyed with criticism about your drinking? Do you sometimes feel guilty about your drinking? Do you sometimes have an eye-opener drink in the morning?

Less than 3 drinks (1 oz. = 1 drink) a day is unlikely to lead to any physical complications. Talk to your pharmacist or M.D. about interactions with medicines. If you are alcoholic, remember you are powerless, and one drink will definitely hurt.

Complications include traffic accidents, depression, family disruption, pneumonia, head and neck cancers, breast cancer, cirrhosis, stomach and esophageal bleeding, memory loss, sudden death, electrolyte disturbances, seizures, pancreatitis, withdrawal reactions, etc. Don't drink during pregnancy. Besides fetal defects, even one drink per week can cause aggressive behavior in the child. Alcohol has also been found to damage the brains of teenagers.

Treatment includes detoxification, Alcoholics Anonymous (no excuses about the time or the group composition) and medicines. One drug called naltrexone (Revia) helps to block opiate receptors in the brain and therefore decreases the pleasurable effects of alcohol. Disulfuram (Antabuse) may decrease drinking because one can develop nausea and severe systemic reactions if alcohol is consumed with this drug. The effects of Antabuse can persist even two weeks after stopping the medication. Other new anticraving drugs such as Acamprosate (Campral) are presently being studied. Treatment of depression and anxiety with agents such as Prozac, Celexa, Zoloft, Paxil and Effexor can be helpful.

The first step must come from you. Admit that you need help! Group support is central for the treatment of this disease.

Allergies

Allergic rhinitis (or allergic nose) affects 10 to 20% of the population. The body's immune system overreacts, and symptoms such as itchy eyes, sneezing and congestion ensue. These symptoms are similar to a cold. Colds, however, are due to viruses and often cause fatigue, green sputum and sometimes fever.

Try to prevent allergies if at all possible. Decrease house dust allergy by reducing the humidity in your house to 50% or less. This will inhibit growth of the dust mite. Wrap your mattress (a big source of dust) in plastic, and obtain an electrostatic filter. A Hepa filter can be very useful in reducing dust. Mold can be reduced by keeping plants out of the house, cleaning up clutter and mopping up any water. Pollen is hard to avoid as it is outside. Air-conditioning can provide relief while you are inside. Also pollen counts rise as the day progresses, hence try going out earlier in the day. Bathe at night to reduce pollen counts on the skin. Cats and dogs can be a real problem. At a minimum, keep them out of the bedroom.

Stick with the less sedating antihistamines such as Claritin, Clarinex, Allegra and Zyrtec. Avoid the over-the-counter, sedating antihistamines since they can cause confusion, driving impairment and drowsiness. Even at bedtime these drugs can cause daytime sleepiness. For instance, diphenhydramine (Benadryl) can impair driving worse than alcohol. This ingredient is found in antiallergy agents and sleep medicine. Nasal steroids, such as Nasonex, Flonase, Rhinocort, etc., actually work the best for moderate to severe nasal allergies. These agents are very well tolerated; however, there may be a mild association with glaucoma. Astelin is a nasal spray that has antihistamine properties. It is particularly useful for relieving nasal stuffiness and works as well as the oral antihistamines. It may cause sedation. If your nose is mainly runny, then consider ipratropium (Atrovent), which helps to dry out the nose.

Butterbur is an alternative herb that may be useful for allergies. Some liver enzyme elevations have been noted. It works as well as the newer antihistamines but must be taken four times a day.

Sometimes allergies will mainly affect the eyes and cause itching and burning. Try Patanol or Zaditor. Both of these agents work quickly and can be used twice daily. Soft contact lenses may absorb the medicine, so wait 10 minutes before putting in your soft contacts.

Alzheimer's

Eighty percent of dementia is due to Alzheimer's, and it is the loss of problem-solving and memory skills that often are not recognized by the affected individual. Usually family members are more aware of such developments than the patient. Five percent at age 70, 20% at age 80 and 50% at age 90 have it. Risk factors for this disease include high cholesterol, family history, and severe head trauma. Often there are deposits in the brain of beta amyloid, an abnormal protein substance that interrupts communication between nerve cells. Genetic testing for the apo E 4 gene is not worthwhile. Even if you have the gene, you may never develop the disease. High cholesterol may cause the production of beta amyloid. A Finnish study showed that an elevated cholesterol (average of 251) and an elevated systolic blood pressure (the upper number) of 160 or greater in midlife predisposed to Alzheimer's as one aged.

Help prevent this disease by taking vitamin B complex. Alzheimer patients have lower levels of this vitamin. Use especially high doses of vitamin B12 (1,000 mcg a day) as it reduces homocysteine. This substance may cause blockages in our vessels and damage nerve cells. (There is less Alzheimer's in women who take conjugated estrogens such as Premarin.) This drug probably helps to improve the short-term memory loss that sometimes occurs around menopause. It does not help treat this disease once it develops. Anti-inflammatories such as ibuprofen or naproxen (watch out for stomach upset or even bleeding ulcers) may also help to prevent this disease. Even low amounts seemed to reduce the incidence of Alzheimer's by 30 to 60%. Such drugs do not help to treat Alzheimer's. A study in *The Journal of the American Medical Association* demonstrated that vitamin C and especially E seemed to be effective in preventing this ailment. Coenzyme Q-10, or Q-Gel (www.DrLipkis.com), can help increase the energy output in our cells, thus possibly reducing neuron loss. Normalizing both the cholesterol and blood pressure is thought to reduce this disease fourfold. The Syst-Eur study showed a 55% reduction in dementia (mostly Alzheimer's) when high blood pressure was controlled. High blood pressure and cholesterol may be responsible for the deposition of beta amyloid, which impairs nerve cell function.

Once Alzheimer's disease develops, ginkgo biloba at 40 mg 3 times a day helped improve memory in these patients. This herb is an anti-inflammatory and also thins the blood. It may delay the progression of the disease by 6 months. Only a standardized extract of this herb, called Ginkgold, was studied. Ginkgo can cause nausea, headache and bleeding. Use with caution if you are taking aspirin or Coumadin. Vitamin E at 1,000 units twice daily may also be useful. Such a dose can help delay institutionalization by 6 months. Once again, this vitamin also thins the blood. Since this disease involves loss of nerve cells, increasing a hormone called acetylcholine can help to stabilize the disease for at least 1 to 2 years. Often behavior will improve with augmentation of this essential hormone for memory. Aricept, Exelon and Reminyl are examples of medicines that increase the amount of this memory hormone. These medicines probably work in dementia due to strokes as well. Sometimes antipsychotics (Risperdal, Zyprexa or Seroquel) and antidepressants are needed to improve behavior. Actually the behavior problems are more frustrating than the memory loss. Caretakers should get help because they are at higher risk for medical problems due to the great stress that this disease causes. The rule of thumb is that you can't take care of others until you first care for yourself. This is one of my rules for life.

Aphthous Ulcers

These ulcers form in the mouth and often are recurrent. The cause is unknown; however, herpes, autoimmune diseases and fungi can mimic these sores. Once a diagnosis is made, treatment can commence. Tetracycline rinses and Apthasol cream can be helpful during an episode.

Propranolol can be very helpful in preventing recurrent episodes. The drug is dosed at 10 mg three times daily for 1 week, then twice daily for a week and finally once daily for 65 days. All patients showed improvement, and 70% had complete clearance of the sores over the 2-to-3-month treatment. Some patients are disease free even three years later.

Asthma

This disease affects 5% of the population and results in cough, wheezing and shortness of breath. The most common aggravating factors include upper respiratory infections, seasonal allergies, exercise and occupational exposures. This is often a genetic condition.

If you have to use a rescue inhaler such as albuterol to open the airways more than three times a week, begin a steroid inhaler under your doctor's guidance. Inhaled steroids can cut the risk of death from asthma by 50%. Regular use of a steroid inhaler can be lifesaving. I stress the word *regular*, since recent discontinuation of inhaled steroids (within 3 months) was implicated in 20 % of asthma deaths. Singulair, a leukotriene inhibitor, works to modulate the immune response in asthma similar to steroid inhalers. It is more convenient (one pill each evening), and can be used in mild asthma. Combining a steroid inhaler with Serevent will work better than just raising the steroid inhaler alone. Serevent works for 12 hours and opens the airways like a rescue inhaler. Serevent will not open the airways for about 20 minutes, so it should not be used as a rescue inhaler. A steroid inhaler reduces the inflammation in the airways and reduces mortality. A good combination inhaler called Advair Discus unites a steroid inhaler (Flovent) with Serevent and is helpful for the treatment of this disease.

Prompt treatment of asthma triggers such as bronchitis, sinusitis or occupational exposures can be useful. If you have exercise-induced asthma, using your rescue inhaler 10 minutes before exercising can help. There are some reports that vitamin C can help exercise-induced asthma as well.

Often emergency room treatment of this disease requires IV steroids and albuterol delivered through a nebulizer. A nebulizer often helps to deliver the medicine to the lungs more effectively than a handheld inhaler. IV magnesium can rapidly improve lung function as well.

Back Pain

This is a very common condition and is the number one cause of disability. Most back pain is due to muscle spasm, degenerative arthritis, nerve pain as a result of a herniated disc (sciatica), spinal stenosis (arthritic spurs pushing on the spinal cord) and stress factors.

Always see your physician first since there are other more serious causes. These include pancreatic cancer, a leaking aortic aneurysm, cancer in the spine, osteoporosis with fractures, kidney disease and infection. Often the latter conditions are worse at rest whereas the common mechanical causes are worse with more activity. Once these serious conditions are ruled out then treatment can commence.

One trial compared massage, acupuncture and placebo therapy. Massage turned out to be the best alternative. Prolonged bed rest or lumbar supports were not useful. Flexeril, a muscle relaxant, has proven useful early in treatment but can cause drowsiness. A supervised exercise program has been helpful in some studies. Chiropractic treatment is also supported by the literature once a diagnosis has been made by your physician. Steroid injections into the spine (epidural injections) have been helpful for herniated discs and arthritis pain relief, but evidence from scientific journals is lacking. Eighty percent of back pain due to the common causes listed above will get better in one month with no care.

MRIs can visualize the back quite well; however, abnormalities can even be seen in normal individuals. An MRI might be useful initially if a serious cause is suspected. Otherwise, treatment with massage, exercises, possibly Flexeril, chiropractic therapy, and time are your best choices. If the pain does not resolve, then an MRI, nerve conduction test and further evaluation are needed.

Cataracts

These opacities form in our lenses with age. Causes include ultraviolet light, steroids, possibly allopurinol (used for gout) and inhaled steroids. Taking daily doses of vitamins E and C may prevent the formation of cataracts. Protect your eyes against UV damage by wearing a brimmed hat and sunglasses. Exposure to UV light is correlated with the development of cataracts.

Cataract removal and the implantation of a new lens are quite successful. Also when surgery is done there is a 50% decrease in subsequent auto accidents.

Chronic Fatigue Syndrome (CFS)

One out of every four individuals suffers from fatigue and 2.5% have chronic fatigue. Some of the more common causes of fatigue include anemia, thyroid disease, depression, sleep disorders, diabetes, cancer, multiple sclerosis, infection and some arthritic conditions.

Unexplained fatigue that occurs for more than 6 months and is not alleviated by rest may fall under the category of chronic fatigue syndrome. Additionally, four or more of the following symptoms should be present: impaired memory, sore throat, muscle aches, headaches, joint aches, tender neck nodes and unrefreshing sleep.

There is no definitive test for CFS. Routine labs in addition to a physical examination can be helpful in eliminating other causes of fatigue. The disease is not caused by the Epstein-Barr virus. This virus does cause mononucleosis and temporary fatigue.

Treatments can include the following:

1) Setting expectations that this disease usually gets better over long periods of time.
2) Treating any concomitant depression may be helpful for concentration and memory problems.
3) Getting adequate sleep at the same bedtime without frequent naps is important.
4) Exercising, such as gentle stretching and walking, helps to improve the functional status.
5) Restoring functional status is very important since there is no cure for the disease. Intravenous immunoglobulins (antibodies), once used in the past, are no longer recommended as they are ineffective.
6) There is scant evidence that some medicines such as Provigil (approved for narcolepsy, a sleep disorder) and amantidine (approved for Parkinson's disease) may be helpful for fatigue in general.

Cirrhosis

Scarring of the liver can be caused by many different ailments such as hepatitis B and C, medications, alcohol, autoimmune disorders, iron/copper overload, etc.

The following preventive measures should be instituted if you have this problem: complete abstinence from alcohol, vaccination against hepatitis A and B, avoidance of iron supplements unless iron loss is noted, a restricted protein diet (see your dietician), endoscopy yearly to make sure that large bleeding veins (varices) aren't forming in the esophagus as a result of the cirrhosis, and regular screening for cancer of the liver with a blood test and ultrasound. People with cirrhosis have a higher incidence of cancer of the liver.

Cold (As in the Common Cold)

There is no cure yet; however, here are a few pointers to help you reduce the nagging symptoms. Avoid antibiotics for the first 7 to 10 days since colds are due to viruses and antibiotics only work on bacteria. Early treatment with antibiotics will only cause bacterial resistance in our population. See your doctor when a cold is prolonged, as it may be a bacterial infection. Usually, this is the case if a cold lasts more than 7 to 10 days. Bacterial infections as opposed to viruses are amenable to antibiotics. Antibiotics can cause yeast infections, allergic reactions, gastrointestinal disturbances, etc. It's safer to receive antibiotics in the office where a physician can diagnose your illness rather than over the phone. Here are a few ideas to help your cold:

1) Try chicken soup (recommended by the Mayo Clinic) as it may reduce the symptoms of a cold.
2) Contac Day and Night may be used for pain and stuffiness.
3) Delsym can be used for cough. This syrup is over the counter and probably works as well as codeine.
4) Echinacea, an herb for boosting the immune system, seems to be helpful in treating colds. Allergic reactions have been reported. Don't take it if you are allergic to ragweed, daisies, etc., since these plants are in the same family as echinacea.
5) Acetaminophen (Tylenol) can be used for fever and pain. A reasonable dosage is 500 mg up to 4 times daily. Ibuprofen may be added to acetaminophen at 2 tablets 4 times daily with food. It also works for pain and fever.

6) Vitamin C may help reduce the duration of symptoms (try 2,000–5,000 mg daily).
7) Zinc lozenges possibly help to reduce the duration of the cold.
8) Drink plenty of fluids. This is an age-old remedy.

All of the above are obtainable over the counter. If you have had your spleen removed or have an immunity problem, it may be wise to start antibiotics sooner.

Finally, a study from Wilkes University in Pennsylvania reveals that sex once to twice a week increases an antibody (immunoglobulin A) that helps to fight upper respiratory infections. Could sex be the best cure for the common cold?

Cold Sores

These are blisters that can form on the lips or in the mouth secondary to the herpes virus. Stress, ultraviolet light and viral infections may cause these sores to appear. The course of these blisters can be shortened by a day or two by taking Valtrex, 2 grams twice a day for one day only.

Common Cardiac Risk Factors

If you can keep your cholesterol under 200, blood pressure 120/80 or less, and not smoke, then it is estimated that you will live an additional 5.8 to 9.5 years. This study analyzed men between the ages of 18 and 59 and women between the ages of 40 and 59.

Diabetes

This disease is the third-leading contributor to death behind obesity and smoking. Type 1 diabetes requires that the patient use insulin because the pancreas cannot produce any. Perhaps this disease is due to an autoimmune problem or a virus. Type 2 diabetes is strongly genetic and is due to an impaired pancreas and insulin resistance. The pancreas may have trouble reducing blood sugar due to impaired insulin secretion. Additionally, the insulin that is produced does not work as well. This is called insulin resistance and usually occurs in diabetics who are overweight.

If your fasting sugar is over 125 or a 2-hour glucose tolerance test shows a sugar over 200, you have diabetes. Have annual eye exams, yearly flu vaccinations, a pneumonia vaccine and examine your feet for cuts. Moisturize your feet daily to avoid cracking and potential infection. Aim for fasting sugars under 110, a 2-hour postprandial sugar under 140, an LDL or bad cholesterol under 100, blood pressure below 130/80 and a hemoglobin A1c (average 3 months of sugars) under 6.5%. Remember to follow an ADA diet (see a dietician) and exercise. These goals are critically important to avoid many of the complications of diabetes such as eye disease, nerve problems and kidney disease. Tighter sugar control can reduce the incidence of these complications by one-third.

Keeping the blood sugar under 110, if you're very sick in the hospital, can reduce serious infections by 50%. Take a 325 mg aspirin daily to help reduce heart attack risk. (Avoid aspirin if you are allergic to it or have stomach problems such as ulcers.) Monitor your sugars daily and have a glucagon injection kit for possible hypoglycemia (low blood sugar). Make sure someone besides yourself knows how to use it just in case you lose consciousness due to a low blood sugar. Glucagon is a hormone that raises blood sugar upon injection.

Additionally, have your doctor look for microalbumin in your urine and begin an ACE inhibitor if small amounts of this protein are found. An ACE inhibitor can reduce protein excretion in the urine, thus relieving some of the adverse effects that diabetes has on the kidneys. ACE inhibitors are marvelous drugs. The HOPE trial showed that people who had coronary artery disease or strokes could effectively reduce future strokes, heart attacks, new onset diabetes and total death rate with the use of Altace, an ACE inhibitor. The optimal dose was 10 mg per day of Altace. These agents also reduce blood pressure and improve survival in heart failure. A good case can be made for placing all diabetics on ACE inhibitors, even if there is no elevation in blood pressure or protein in the urine.

ARBs are another class of drugs that have been proven to reduce protein in the urine and protect the kidneys. Examples include Cozaar, Diovan, Avapro and Atacand. Cozaar has even delayed the onset of kidney failure. It is not clear at this time if ACE inhibitors will also prevent kidney failure. An ARB medicine such as Cozaar is a first-line choice in type 2 diabetics who have protein in the urine.

If your sugars before meals appear well controlled (under 120) and your Hemoglobin A1c is elevated, try checking a sugar 2 hours after a meal. If it is greater than 140, further treatment is needed. The Hemoglobin A1c is a valuable assessment of sugar control. This test measures the average sugar over a 3-month time period. An elevated value implies that the sugar control is less than optimal.

Statins, a class of cholesterol-lowering agents (Lipitor, Zocor, Lescol, Pravachol, etc.), may actually help to reduce the incidence of diabetes by 30%, perhaps by helping our insulin to work better. This effect was specifically shown with Pravachol. This drug has also markedly reduced protein excretion by the kidneys.

Lantus, a once-a-day, long-acting insulin, provides a steady release of insulin. It is convenient and results in fewer episodes of hypoglycemia. This insulin is clear, may sting with injection and should not be combined with other insulin types.

Disintegrator Plus, a portable needle disposal kit, costs around $100 and looks like a pencil sharpener. Each needle is placed in the hole of the machine. The needle is heated until a small ball of metal comes out. The nub can then be disposed.

Finally, with diabetes, be sure to exercise and see a registered dietician. Regular exercise and weight loss can reduce the new onset of diabetes by 67% in people who are already borderline for this disease. (See Appendix A for more details concerning diabetes.)

Exercise

Sedentary lifestyle might indeed be the biggest risk factor for heart disease in the USA! More than 75% of people fail to do one vigorous activity per week.

Aerobic exercise 3 times a week for 11 to 25 minutes can reduce heart attacks by 33%. Walking 2 miles daily reduced mortality by 50%. In another study, exercise may help to extend lifespan by 5 to 10 years by lowering the rates of heart attacks, cancer (colon, breast and prostate), depression and anxiety, diabetes, osteoporosis, obesity and insomnia. The immune system may also be enhanced. Walking seems to be just as beneficial as aerobic activity.

Here is a simple formula to calculate your appropriate heart rate during exercise. Take 220 minus your age (this is your maximal heart rate) and multiply it by 70%. If you are 50 years old, your safe heart rate might be around 125. If you're out of shape, aim for 60%, and if you are in excellent shape, go for 80 % of your maximal heart rate. Always check with your health provider.

A simple routine might include stretching for 5 minutes, warming up for 2 minutes, fast walking with coordinated arm swinging for 20 minutes, cooling down for 2 minutes, using free weights for 15 minutes and stretching for 5 minutes. Always drink plenty of water. For vigorous exercise consider replacing fluid losses with Gatorade, since it contains salt, sugar and water. Marathon runners are prone to low salt levels; hence both salt and water must be replaced. Low salt levels can lead to brain damage.

Vigorous exertion, for example, snow shoveling, may trigger sudden death by promoting coronary plaque rupture. In other words, cholesterol plaque in a heart vessel can break open and bleed. The blood can then clot and block blood flow within the vessel. Once the heart muscle is unable to receive blood flow, a heart attack may ensue. Regular exercise done in moderation can reduce overall risk of nonsudden cardiac death. Don't be a weekend warrior. More sudden deaths occur after vigorous workouts, if done once a week or less. Once again, regular exercise is key. Vince Lombardi, the legendary Green Bay Packers coach, said that exercise is about 90% inspiration and 10% perspiration. Your desire will play a critical role. Saying that you have a treadmill in the basement or that you belong to a health club doesn't gain you any brownie points in my book. Taking action is key. One study shows that incorporating exercise into your activities of daily living can be helpful. For instance, park your car further from work, take the stairs instead of the elevator, get up from your computer station every hour, etc. Make exercise fun and not a chore!

Fibromyalgia

This is a syndrome seen mainly in women and characterized by painful trigger points at multiple sites, headache, fatigue and insomnia. Other arthritic diseases must be excluded.

Treatment includes low-impact aerobics, stretching and light weights. Exercises that might be considered include yoga, tai chi and swimming. Anti-inflammatories do not help very often. Tricyclic antidepressants such as Elavil can be helpful for sleep and relieving pain. SSRI antidepressants such as Prozac, Zoloft, and Paxil can also be tried for pain relief and any associated depression. Neurontin, which helps with nerve pain, may be useful in this condition. Ultram can sometimes work by increasing serotonin and norepinephrine (like adrenaline) in the brain. There is a very low rate of addiction with this agent. Natural remedies may include SAMe (don't combine with antidepressants), and possibly Guaifenasin. The latter, at 600 mg three times a day, may help to excrete phosphate from the muscles and reduce pain. Guaifenasin is in over-the-counter cough syrups, but may be too sugary. Try the prescription version, called Humibid.

Gambling

About 1 to 2% of the nation are pathologic gamblers. Just like alcoholism, this problem can be socially devastating. Antidepressants such as Paxil at 60 mg per day may be helpful. This drug will work especially well if the gambling is accompanied by depression. Mood stabilizers such as Depakote and lithium can help decrease the gambling urge, especially if the person is bipolar. Naltrexone, a drug used for alcoholics, can also be useful. Group support and psychotherapy may prove beneficial as well.

Hepatitis C

This virus affects 4 million people in the USA, and most people have no symptoms. Eighty-five percent go on to develop chronic disease that can lead to scarring or cirrhosis of the liver. It is the number one cause of liver transplantation. Risk factors include blood transfusion prior to 1992, needlestick injury, elevated liver function, intravenous drug use, possibly cocaine snorting, body piercing/tattooing and being in prison.

Hepatitis C may also be transmitted by sexual

intercourse and from mother to child during birth. Transmission of the virus by these routes is less common.

Get tested by your physician if you have done any of the high-risk behaviors indicated above. This disease commonly mimics rheumatoid arthritis. (Joint pains commonly occur.) Remember to get vaccinated against hepatitis A and B and never drink alcohol if you have this disease. In other words, the goal is avoiding any additional liver injury. Rebetol (ribavirin) with PEG-Intron (interferon a) is an effective, antiviral combination for treating this disease. PEG-Intron is a long-acting interferon that is injected only once a week. This sustained-release form of the drug is likely more effective than the plain antiviral drug, interferon.

HIV

As of 2001 about 36 million people worldwide are living with the AIDS virus. The most common mode of spread is illicit, intravenous drug use. Heterosexual spread is the next most common way, and transmission via this route is rapidly increasing. Male-to-male spread has decreased over the last several years. Most new cases are now occurring in Hispanics and African Americans.

Consider getting an HIV test if you have used intravenous drugs, have had a homosexual experience, have had multiple sex partners, have been diagnosed with a sexually transmitted disease, or have a disease that can signal HIV infection (such as unexplained recurrent vaginal yeast infections, oral yeast infection, shingles, lymph nodes, pneumonias, etc.).

The first stage of HIV infection is called the acute retroviral syndrome. Symptoms are often flulike and may include fever, rash, lymph node enlargement, sore throat and muscle aches. If such symptoms occur in the setting of high-risk behavior, blood testing (HIV-RNA virus load) should be done. Pregnant women should be tested for HIV since AZT therapy can reduce mother-baby transmission from 30% to 8%.

Today HIV infection is treated once helper T cells (the immune-fighting cells) fall below 350/cc. Many drugs, called antiretroviral therapy, are used to treat this disease. The prognosis for HIV survival used to be 10 to 12 years, but now it is estimated that infected individuals will live 30 to 35 years. Compliance with taking multiple medications and worldwide distribution of these life-saving drugs are essential if successful treatment is to occur. An AIDS vaccine is presently under development. Even if it is partially effective, such a vaccine can have an enormous impact on this disease.

Hypertension

Add several years to your life by keeping your blood pressure under 140/90. The ideal reading is 120/80. Even high-normal readings, 130–139/85–89, may be associated with increased risk of cardiovascular disease. If you have diabetes, strokes or heart disease, keep your blood pressure under 130/80. If you have kidney disease, consider keeping the pressure under 125/75.

Hypertension is the silent killer. Control the pressure and subsequently reduce strokes by 40%, heart attacks by 20%, and decrease kidney disease and blindness as well. Lifestyle changes that can help include increasing potassium, calcium and magnesium intake, restricting salt, losing weight, exercising, taking coenzyme Q-10 (my favorite brand is Q-Gel), increasing fruits, vegetables, and grains, and having no more than 2 alcoholic beverages daily.

Resperate, an over-the-counter breathing device in the form of a CD player, can lower blood pressure by 10 to 15 points. The device helps you to slow breathing rates down to 10 breaths per minute and should be used 3 to 4 times per week for 15 minutes. The device is expensive but in the long run, it's cheaper than medication.

Forty percent of patients have elevated readings at the office and should do home blood pressure monitoring, especially in the morning when pressure is the highest. Aim for home readings below 135/85. Another more accurate way to measure pressure out of the office is to wear a 24-hour ambulatory blood pressure monitor. Taking a portable unit with you during the day automatically measures your blood pressure over a 24-hour time period. Hypertension in the doctor's office may mean that you are having hypertension on the job or under stress. If the pressure is normal at home and elevated elsewhere, there still may be some additional risk to the heart and brain.

Have your eye doctor check your retina. This is the membrane in the back of your eye that allows you to see. If the retinal arteries show hypertensive changes, then the blood pressure should be treated. Evidently in this scenario, eye damage implies that your pressure should be better controlled because arterial disease is occurring as a result of hypertension.

Sometimes the cheapest agents are the best for treatment. Thiazide diuretics probably reduce the risk of stroke more than other agents; however, they may lower potassium and raise sugar slightly. This drug also retains calcium, which may be good for osteoporosis. Another class of medications called ACE inhibitors can be helpful. Altace, a specific ACE inhibitor, can reduce stroke, heart attacks and new-onset diabetes. These drugs probably have an antiatherogenic effect, thus reducing plaque in our arteries. Other tissue ACE inhibitors that may have similar properties include Aceon, Lotensin, Accupril and Mavik. A third class of blood pressure medications is called ARBs. These agents include Cozaar, Diovan, Avapro, Tevetin, Micardis, Atacand and Benicar. They are also effective medicines and have lower side effects compared to other antihypertensive agents. ARBs are also more expensive. Beta blockers are another class of drugs that can lower blood pressure. Examples include Toprol XL, Tenormin, Inderal and Coreg. These agents may be especially useful if hypertension is accompanied by heart failure or coronary disease. Alpha blockers such as Cardura should not be used first line for the treatment of hypertension. Such drugs may cause shortness of breath.

Irritable Bowel Syndrome (IBS)

This common bowel problem is defined by at least 12 weeks of abdominal pain in the last 12 months. Two other features include alterations in stool form or frequency and pain relieved by a bowel movement. One may also have constipation, diarrhea or both.

It is important to exclude colitis, tumors, bacterial overgrowth, malabsorption and lactose intolerance. These diseases may imitate irritable bowel syndrome and are also treatable. Foods that may aggravate IBS include alcohol, grape and apple juice, sorbitol (found in chewing gum and candy), bananas, chocolate, cabbage, carrots, brussels sprouts, pretzels, bagels, caffeine, broccoli, dairy products, large meals and high-fat foods.

If you have primarily constipation, you may benefit from increasing your fiber with Metamucil and various high-fiber foods. Zelnorm, at 6 mg twice a day, can be effective for patients with irritable bowel who primarily have constipation. It is approved only for women. Neomycin, an antibiotic, at 500 mg twice daily for 10 days may be helpful. This drug may kill bacteria that may aggravate this disease. Further research is needed regarding neomycin's efficacy in IBS. Probiotics may also help to reduce symptoms of IBS. These agents contain specific bacteria such as Lactobacillus and Bifidobacterium. The latter bacteria seems to work particularly well in IBS. Peppermint oil in capsule form 3 times a day may help to relieve constipation and spasm. (Look for 2 to 4 ml of peppermint oil in each enteric coated capsule.)

For predominantly diarrhea Bentyl, Levsin, Prilosec and antidepressants may be helpful. These same medicines may also be helpful with constipation as well. Lotronex is approved on a limited basis to help with the predominantly diarrhea type of irritable bowel.

Macular Degeneration

This disease is the leading cause of blindness in the elderly. Smoking is the only known risk factor. Painless loss of central vision is the main symptom. There are two types: wet and dry. The wet type is often associated with hemorrhage and can be treated with laser or photodynamic therapy (a laser treatment after a chemical is injected, which helps target the laser toward the central vision).

Lutein, an antioxidant found in green leafy vegetables, might help to prevent this disease. Coenzyme Q-10 may also be helpful. Evidence with both these agents is scanty. Patients who take statin medications to lower cholesterol seem to have a lower rate of developing this disease.

A trial in the U.S. showed that patients with macular degeneration can reduce progression by 25% by taking a vitamin containing beta carotene, vitamin E, zinc, and vitamin C called Ocuvite-PreserVision by Bausch and Lomb.

Migraine

Twenty million Americans have it and the cause is unknown. Migraines seem to originate in the brain stem and activate like a spark plug. There is usually a family history in 80% of patients with migraines. If you are having the worst headache of your life or if your usual migraine headaches are suddenly worsening, a CAT scan and possibly a spinal tap are indicated. These tests help rule out more serious causes of headaches such as a brain hemorrhage, tumor or stroke.

Characteristics of migraine headaches include nausea, sensitivity to light, sound or smells, and pounding nature. Often the headaches are worse during menstrual periods and occur on one side (not always). Migraine headaches may also be worse during sex and exertion. Sometimes visual and motor disturbances occur before the onset of the migraine.

If you are having more than 3 headaches per month, try a preventive medication such as Propranolol, Depakote, Neurontin, Elavil, Zestril, Atacand, Vioxx plus Singulair, or Verapamil. Riboflavin at 400 mg daily (vitamin B2) can work in 50% after 3 months. Coenzyme Q-10 at 100 mg daily can also be effective within the same time period.

Acute headaches may be relieved by the triptans (Imitrex, Maxalt, Zomig, Axert, etc.). Don't use these agents if there is a history of heart disease or you are at increased cardiac risk, such as from smoking. Anti-inflammatories like Excedrin, Motrin and Aleve may be helpful. Nondrug therapy includes avoiding alcohol, eating meals on time, maintaining the same sleep-wake cycle, biofeedback, massage, ice packs and stress reduction. Magnesium and feverfew are alternative therapies.

Rebound headaches are common with the frequent use of nasal decongestants, aspirin, caffeine, acetaminophen, Fiorinal, codeine and even the triptans. Avoiding frequent use of these medications is essential. Your doctor can also try Amerge (a triptan medicine with perhaps less rebound), Zanaflex (a muscle relaxant) plus Vioxx or Celebrex. These agents can help with pain and are associated with much less rebound. In other words daily use, for example, of Excedrin can result in more headaches as this medicine withdraws from your system. Zanaflex and muscle massage therapy for chronic daily headaches that are not rebound in nature can be helpful.

Finally, sinus headaches, which people often note, might not really exist. Many neurologists now believe that such headaches are migraine in nature.

Obesity

This condition is primarily a genetic disease (70%). It is defined as a body mass index of 30 or above. The body mass index (BMI) is better at predicting what a healthy body weight is. Please see Appendix B. The BMI correlates directly with the risk of heart disease and stroke. This is especially true if this index is 30 or greater.

Obesity is associated with diabetes, hypertension, premature death, gallstones, osteoarthritis, coronary disease, sleep apnea and some cancers. A 10% weight loss can have a profound effect on your health.

Exercising, even if you don't lose weight, will lengthen your life. Keep a food diary, see your dietician, exercise to music, videotapes, etc.—make it fun! Get motivated with a pedometer that measures the number of steps you take each day. Figure out your baseline number of steps, and then each week gradually increase the distance. Also, stop eating when you are full, don't shop when you are hungry, avoid cues that are associated with eating (TV, newspapers, etc.). Ask yourself the following question: Am I eating because I'm hungry or am I eating to fulfill another need? Remember to drink 8 glasses of water a day. If you are stressed or depressed, have this treated first by your physician and therapist. Also set appropriate expectations—a 10% weight loss maintained for a year or more will help improve your health immensely and is a barometer of success.

My favorite nutritional plan is the Mediterranean diet (see Chapter 4). Low-carbohydrate, high-protein diets certainly work in many, but the consumption of fruits and vegetables is decreased, and we do not know the long-term side effects. Take a multiple vitamin with these low-carbohydrate nutritional plans and make sure your doctor rechecks your uric acid and your cholesterol profile. (These lab values may rise on this type of dietary plan.) These diets probably work because the higher protein intake makes you feel full and fewer calories are generally consumed. In general, cholesterol decreases on this regimen. One reduces carbohydrates by decreasing white bread, potatoes, corn, fruits, certain desserts, vegetables, pasta, etc. *Sugar Busters* and *Atkins' New Diet Revolution* are excellent resources.

Meridia helps to decrease your appetite while eating. The drug can raise blood pressure and heart rate. This medicine may interact with antidepressants that increase serotonin. The drug does not cause heart valve damage like the old combo of phentermine and fenfluramine. One usually takes 10 to 15 mg per daily.

Xenical blocks 30% of fat from being absorbed. This may result in diarrhea and stool incontinence. If you restrict your fat intake and take 12 grams of psyllium at bedtime, side effects can be reduced. Xenical can also reduce the chances of developing diabetes beyond diet and exercise alone. This medicine is taken three times daily with any meal that contains fat.

Both of these drugs are costly, have some side effects and result in a 5 to 10 percent weight loss. Green tea capsules, with minimal caffeine, may increase thermogenesis (heat production) and help you lose weight. Preliminary studies show that Wellbutrin, an antidepressant, Topomax, an antiseizure/migraine drug, and Glucophage, an antidiabetic agent, may help with weight loss.

Don't take products with ephedra and caffeine, as excess cardiovascular deaths have occurred. If you are taking such a product (which I am against), make sure that there is no more than 25 mg of total ephedra alkaloids in each serving (maximum of 100 mg per day). Conjugated linoleic acid (CLA) at 3 grams a day may help to regulate body fat by reducing fat and increasing muscle mass. Chromium picolinate, at 200 mcg daily, may help to convert fat to muscle. More studies are forthcoming. Other herbal/vitamin weight loss aids include Hydroxycitrate (found in Citrimax, Citrilean, Diet Fuel, Herbalife), which may inhibit fat production but no effect on weight has been demonstrated. Bitter orange and country mallow (heartleaf) are also stimulants and similar to ephedra. Avoid them. Taking 7-keto DHEA may boost metabolism and result in weight loss, but long-term side effects are not known. I urge you to check the labels on these weight-loss formulas.

Here is a sample plan for losing weight based upon recent data:

1) You must be motivated to succeed. If you are depressed, anxious or have a family history of abuse, address these issues first with your therapist and physician.
2) Secondary causes of being overweight are rare but may need investigation. Conditions that may contribute to obesity include thyroid diseases, polycystic ovary syndrome, Cushing's syndrome (an overproduction of steroids in the body) and certain medications such as antidepressants, antipsychotics and corticosteroids.
3) Mark a day on your calendar and focus on that particular day. Get the junk food out of the house. Make sure that your family knows and supports your efforts. If your spouse does the cooking, you will need to enlist his or her help.
4) Make up a grid and split it into three columns. Label the three columns *time, exercise,* and *food.* Every time you eat, mark what foods you have consumed in the appropriate column. Do the same with the exercise

column. This concept is called "stimulus control." Such feedback will help to keep you on track.

5) Increase your dairy intake. Adding several servings a day of yogurt, skim milk, low-fat cheese, etc., helped dieters lose 70% more weight than nondairy consumers. Calcium will not only help keep your bones strong, but it tells the fat cell to burn fat rather than store it. Milk without exercise and diet doesn't accomplish much. Add 3 to 4 servings of dairy a day with a nutritional plan and you've got something!

6) Limit alcohol to one glass per day. While this beverage in moderation is healthy for the heart and possibly cancer prevention, it still has plenty of calories. For example, the consumption of 3,500 calories will cause you to gain about 1 pound. Each alcoholic beverage contains about 250 calories. If you have 3 drinks daily, then you are consuming about 750 additional calories daily. If you decrease your consumption to 1 drink per day, then you are consuming 3,500 calories less per week. Theoretically, you should then lose 1 pound per week and help your heart.

7) It is so important to consult with a dietician. Such a skilled professional can give you the specifics of the diet that you wish to pursue. Sixty percent of our nation is overweight despite all the new books, technology, fads, etc. Weight loss can be accomplished, but why not partner with a dietician.

8) If you desire to follow a low-carbohydrate and high-protein program, you will need to avoid the more sugary foods. Such foods include puffed rice, corn flakes, maltose, white rice, 40% bran flakes, white and whole-wheat bread, carrots, shredded wheat, apricots, honey, brown rice, corn chips, oat bran, bananas, white potato, honey, corn, raisins, papaya, white or whole-wheat spaghetti noodles, macaroni, beets, apple juice, rye (whole meal or pumpernickel), applesauce, kidney beans, oatmeal cookies and mangos. Low-sugar foods

include frozen peas, yams, custard, barley, sweet potato, grapes, oranges, grapefruit, navy beans, sponge cake, rye (whole grain), orange juice, lentils, plums, cherries, peaches, yogurt, milk, tomatoes, apples, strawberries, pears, soybeans, peanuts, broccoli, eggplant, lettuce, spinach, green beans, asparagus, cauliflower, cucumber and cabbage.

9) On a low-carbohydrate, high-protein diet, you lose weight because you are consuming fewer calories. The higher intake of protein may result in feeling fuller. You do not burn more fat. Much of our population seems to crave carbohydrates, hence there is a role for this diet. Here are some examples for the three meals. Breakfast: a 6-egg omelet (containing 2 eggs and 4 egg whites), 1 piece of fruit and 2 slices of whole-grain rye. Lunch: 4 ounces of tuna, 1 tablespoon of mayonnaise, 2 rye crackers, 1 piece of fruit, 3 cups of lettuce, and 2 tablespoons of low-fat Italian dressing. Dinner: 6 ounces of chicken breast, 1 large sweet potato and 1 cup of low-glycemic (less sugary) vegetables. Feel free to have a handful of nuts for a snack. Nuts, similar to fish, contain omega-3 fatty acids and likely reduce heart attacks and sudden death. The most difficult part of this dietary plan is sticking to it for a long period of time.

10) Contrary to popular belief, low-carbohydrate diets do indeed lower LDL or bad cholesterol and raise HDL or good cholesterol. The main side effects are constipation and halitosis (bad breath).

11) Low-fat diets work in many individuals and should be discussed with your dietician.

12) Don't skip meals. The body's metabolism will slow down if the "engine" doesn't get fuel. A couple of snacks per day are worthwhile, too.

13) Drink 8 glasses of water a day. I question the proof of this statement, but it's certainly not harmful. Additionally, you will feel fuller.

14) Exercise is essential. Even if you are overweight, exercise helps to protect you against health problems as a result of your weight. Yes, it is better to be overweight and exercise than to be a normal-weight "couch potato." Make exercise fun. Walk with a friend, take a yoga class, go out dancing, get a regular weekly tennis game, listen to good music while on the treadmill, and finally, enlist a personal trainer. A trainer can help with motivation and organize a safe program for you. Longer exercise periods will help you to lose more weight because you are burning more calories. Your body can continue to burn more calories up to 12 hours after exercise!

15) Avoid the cues that condition you to eat more or make improper choices. Possible cues include card games, TV, movies, bars, certain beverages, the newspaper and stress. Also, avoid shopping when you're hungry. Put the smart choices in your refrigerator. View food as fuel needed to survive rather than as a party in your mouth. If you are not hungry, don't eat! Keep in touch with your feelings. Easing stress with food feels different than quelling hunger. Consider eating a meal while you stand. Make the "party" less pleasurable.

16) Alternative supplements that may be helpful include CLA and a weight-loss formula by Physician Nutraceutical. CLA appears safe, and preliminary data is promising for weight loss in human beings. The Weight Loss Formula contains chitosan, which may help to absorb fat (avoid if allergic to shellfish). Other ingredients include chromium picolinate (perhaps mild weight loss by burning sugar), green tea (increases body metabolism), Avantra Z (stimulates beta 3 receptors in fat cells, which might help with fat burning). This fine product can be purchased with a money-back guarantee by calling 1-866-775-7628. Realize that both standard medicine and alternative medicine are only possible aids in losing weight. Further alternative medicines are discussed above.

17) Standard medicines approved for long-term weight loss include Meridia and Xenical and are discussed above. Phentermine is a stimulant that is approved for short-term use in weight loss. This drug may increase blood pressure and pulse rate.

18) Above all, have faith in yourself. Sure, there are genetic overrides that do play a significant role. Enlist a weight loss team, which may consist of family, caring friends, a dietician, an interested physician and a trainer. Alcoholics don't quit by themselves. Food addiction is no different. With the proper attitude, support team, exercise and eating you can do it!

Osteoarthritis

The loss of cartilage, the lubricating substance between bones, leads to "wear and tear" arthritis, or osteoarthritis. Common contributing factors include obesity, female sex, age, trauma and inflammation. The following are standard and alternative measures to help this most common disease:

1) Exercise can prove helpful to the affected joint if done in moderation. Gentle stretching, walking, biking on low resistance and swimming may have a positive effect on osteoarthritis. Physical therapy may also be useful since the exercises can be individualized.

2) Tylenol is generally safe, if the daily dose is under 4,000 mg per day. Tylenol Arthritis contains 650 mg of Tylenol in a sustained-release form. One to two pills three times daily could prove useful. Higher doses may affect the liver adversely.

3) Anti-inflammatory agents can decrease the pain in this disease. Cox-2 inhibitors are anti-inflammatories that have many fewer gastrointestinal side effects than standard anti-inflammatories. Such drugs include Bextra, Celebrex and Vioxx. Rarely, kidney and liver side effects can be associated with these medicines.

4) Vitamin C doesn't prevent this disease but it can slow progression by threefold according to Framingham data. Vitamin D may have the same effect as vitamin C.

5) Glucosamine and chondroitin have about the same effects as anti-inflammatories but with fewer adverse reactions. Additionally, it may take 2 to 8 weeks to see whether or not this alternative medicine works. Glucosamine probably is the most active ingredient. At 1,500 mg per day this over-the-counter medicine may also help to prevent progression of disease. Glucosamine may affect your sugar level. Diabetics especially should be aware of this possible side effect. Some manufacturers will combine glucosamine with chondroitin and MSM to achieve optimal pain relief. It is not known whether chondroitin and MSM add any additional therapeutic value to glucosamine.

6) Doxycycline is an antibiotic that helps to prevent cartilage breakdown in animals. Human studies are already under way for this common antibiotic.

7) Synvisc is a honeylike substance that is approved for osteoarthritis of the knee. It is given in a series of three injections and can significantly decrease pain. Usually the effects of the drug will last for 6 to 18 months. Redness at the site of the injection is a common side effect.

8) An avocado and soybean mixture helped to decrease pain and disability due to osteoarthritis. In another study progression of the disease was reduced as well. Further investigation will be needed.

9) Strengthening the underlying bone beneath the cartilage may be helpful. Therefore medicines used to treat osteoporosis may help to treat osteoarthritis. At this time studies with Actonel (builds bone) are under way.

10) Steroid injections may provide temporary relief of osteoarthritis. Often such injections are reserved for when a joint, such as the knee, suddenly becomes more painful.

Osteoporosis

This is a common problem in menopausal and postmenopausal women. A low bone density can result in hip, spine and wrist fractures· Osteoporosis kills more women at age 75 than breast and pelvic cancers combined. When an older person fractures a hip, there is a 30 to 40% death rate at the end of one year. Often serious complications arise from such a fracture. Blood clots and infection are just a couple of serious consequences after a hip replacement.

Risk factors for osteoporosis include a family history, menopause, blonde hair and blue eyes, anorexia, alcohol, smoking, diabetes, rheumatoid arthritis, inflammatory bowel disease, lack of vitamin D, hyperthyroidism, parathyroid disease and malabsorption.

Help prevent this disease by doing weight-bearing exercises and adding calcium to the food you eat. (A cup of calcium-fortified orange juice, a cup of milk and a cup of yogurt each contains about 300 mg of calcium.) An additional 200 mg generally is obtained from your diet. Aim for 1,000 mg of calcium daily if you are premenopausal, and 1,500 mg of calcium if you are postmenopausal. Men can take between 1,000 and 1,500 mg of calcium daily. A good and cheap source of calcium is Tums 500. Each chewable tablet contains 500 mg of calcium. Viactiv, a chewable chocolate calcium, also contains 500 mg of calcium and is available over the counter. Both Tums 500 and Viactiv must be taken with food in divided doses for better absorption. Citracal, another form of calcium, may be taken with or without food. Vitamin D is also important. Older folks derive significant benefits from vitamin D, including decreased falls and increased muscle strength. This likely results from increased muscle uptake of calcium, which helps the muscle contract. Vitamin D may be obtained by going out into sunlight or by taking a multiple vitamin. An optimal amount of vitamin D daily is 400 to

800 units (see Appendix H). Finally, remember to get screened for osteoporosis around menopause. Fosamax, Actonel, Miacalcin and Evista can help prevent and treat osteoporosis. Estrogen is approved for the prevention of this disease. Accurate screening for osteoporosis can occur by scanning the finger, wrist or heel. A dexa scan is much more expensive but directly screens the hip and spine. Estrogen therapy and Fosamax increase bone density in the spine and the hip whereas Evista and Miacalcin increase bone density in the spine only. Fosamax and Actonel come in a once-weekly formulation and are members of the same class of drugs called biphosphonates. Fosamax has more studies with regard to efficacy in osteoporosis, but unlike Actonel, remains in the bones for at least a decade. Evista and estrogen can slightly increase the chance of blood clots. Evista probably decreases the risk of breast cancer and reduces CRP, a marker for increased heart attacks. Estrogen plus Fosamax can increase bone density more than estrogen alone. Forteo (human parathyroid hormone) is an injectable drug approved for osteoporosis. It is injected under the skin daily and can be used to treat women who are at high risk for fractures.

Estrogen is approved for the prevention but not treatment of osteoporosis. If it is combined with progesterone, the risks of breast cancer, stroke and heart attack increase. Estrogen should not be given first line for osteoporosis unless prominent menopausal symptoms are also present. Symptoms may include hot flashes, mood swings, night sweats, vaginal dryness, etc. (Please see Appendix C for more information regarding osteoporosis.)

Parkinson's Disease

This neurological disorder mainly occurs in the elderly. Fifteen percent of the U.S. population between 65 and 75 has this disease. Fifty percent of the elderly 85 and older develop Parkinson's.

When 80% of the nerve cells regulating movement degenerate, this disorder occurs. The cause is unknown in most patients, but sometimes this disease may be precipitated by infection, drugs, toxic exposures and vascular problems. The end result is a lack of dopamine, which is necessary for movement.

Symptoms may include a resting "pill rolling" tremor, little or no arm swing, masklike face, stooped posture and poor balance. Progression of symptoms is quite variable.

Treatment revolves around replacing dopamine. Levodopa should not be used initially because after a few years of use, excessive movements called dyskinesias may occur. It is usually better to begin with medications that are dopamine agonists. Such agents include Permax, Parlodel, Requip and Mirapex. These may cause sudden sleep attacks. Levodopa is often added when the dopamine agonists no longer work. Comtan may be added to levodopa to help it last longer and reduce dyskinesias. Seroquel or Zyprexa may be useful in reducing hallucinations, which are common with this disease.

Physical therapy can help with the poor balance that often occurs with this ailment. Additionally, social services may be needed for both the caregiver and the patient. Depression and dementia may accompany Parkinson's, and the strain on the caregiver can resemble that of stress on caregivers of those with Alzheimer's disease.

Deep brain stimulation may be helpful in reducing medication for this disease and improving quality of life. A probe is inserted on both sides of the brain where Parkinson's disease occurs. These electrodes are connected to a pulse generator under the skin. This is like a pacemaker for the brain. The patient can control the amount of current that this pacemaker generates. This concept is a definite breakthrough for Parkinson's disease.

Coenzyme Q-10 at higher doses (1,200 mg daily) can help slow this disease by 44%. Call 1-866-775-7628.

Physical Exam

Have one regularly to detect the silent problems such as cancer, high blood pressure, diabetes, high cholesterol, coronary disease, etc. Let's face it, how can we enjoy our lives maximally without health? It would be a shame to develop a new idea at work and then have a heart attack due to silent uncontrolled blood pressure. Yes, I can be your doctor in your house but no resource takes the place of a thorough history and physical exam done by a skilled health provider.

Pulmonary Embolus

Blood clots can be thrown to the lungs and commonly cause shortness of breath, fast heart rate and chest pain. This problem probably contributes to 15 to 30% of all deaths. The source of these clots often is the legs and thighs. The risk factors for clots in the lower extremities include immobility (hospitalizations, long plane flights or recent surgery), hereditary and acquired clotting disorders (such as cancer) and trauma to the legs. Medications such as estrogen and Evista can also increase the risks for clots.

A CAT scan of the chest and a special lung scan can be used to diagnose this disorder. If the diagnosis is not made clear with these tests, an angiogram may need to be done. This test consists of injecting dye into the lung vessels to visualize any clots. Alternatively, if a CAT scan of the lungs and an ultrasound of the leg veins show no clots, the likelihood of dying from a pulmonary embolus is quite low. Finally, if a special blood test called a D-dimer is less than 500 mg/ml (done by the Elisa method in the lab), the odds are that you do not have a blood clot. The D-dimer test measures clot-breakdown products and is helpful in excluding a blood clot. This blood test still needs further study.

Treatment of a blood clot in the lung usually involves two blood thinners that are used in sequence. First heparin shots are given, then Coumadin, an oral blood thinner, is administered. Often the Coumadin is given for at least 6 months. Periodic blood monitoring of this medication is needed. Longer periods of treatment with Coumadin may be required if the underlying risk factor for clots is still present.

Most older patients that are hospitalized should receive preventive heparin shots (such as Lovenox) daily to prevent blood clots from forming in the legs. Compressive leg and thigh stockings can also be useful in prevention. Immobility is a significant risk factor for clot formation.

Rheumatoid Arthritis

This is a genetic disease predominantly affecting females between the ages of 25 and 50. The diagnosis is made if the individual develops four or more of the following seven symptoms: early morning stiffness lasting more than 6 weeks, arthritis in 3 or more joints lasting longer than 6 weeks, hand and wrist involvement, symmetrical arthritis, skin nodules (rheumatoid nodules), bony x-ray changes and a positive rheumatoid factor (a lab test for rheumatoid arthritis). This disease probably occurs due to an overactive immune system. Most of the drugs used to treat the disease help to suppress one's own immune reaction. Hydroxychloroquine or sulfasalazine can be used for initial therapy in mild rheumatoid arthritis. A drug called methotrexate (liver and lung monitoring is needed) also can be used initially to slow down moderate to severe disease. With this ailment, the methotrexate is often dosed weekly, not daily. Joint damage often occurs in the first two years of onset. A disease—modifying agent (methotrexate, hydroxychloroquine or sulfasalazine) should be initiated within the first three months of the onset of this disease. Anti-inflammatories can help to relieve pain but do not decrease disease progression. Interleukin-1 and tumor necrosis factor are immune factors in our body that can aggravate this disease. Agents such as Arava, Enbrel and Remicade are expensive, injectable medicines that can block tumor necrosis factor and reduce the progression of rheumatoid arthritis. Kineret blocks the effect of interleukin-1 and is equally as effective as the previous three listed agents. Experimental therapies include fish oil, tetracyline (an antibiotic) and plamapheresis (removal of antibodies from the blood).

Sinusitis

Eighty percent of colds are accompanied by sinusitis, but usually this condition is treated with antibiotics if it doesn't go away on its own in 10 to 14 days. Often sinusitis is caused by the pneumococcus bacterium. The sinuses are unable to empty during an infection because the tubes draining them become clogged. Other causes of sinusitis include allergies, structural causes (polyps, deviated septum), smoking, IgA antibody deficiency, fungus, cystic fibrosis, etc. Headaches (especially with bending over), foul taste, purulent nasal drainage and fever are common symptoms.

Treatment should include an antibiotic for 2 weeks. Nasal steroids help to reduce symptoms more quickly and also help to reduce recurrences of acute sinusitis. Chronic sinusitis gives low-grade symptoms such as headache and yellow/green drainage that may go on for months. Treatment often includes antibiotics for a duration of 3 to 6 weeks. SinuNEB is a nebulizer that delivers antibiotics to the sinuses in the form of an aerosol spray. Each treatment takes around 10 minutes, and the device is usually used twice daily for 1 to 3 weeks. This treatment is likely more effective than oral antibiotics.

Smallpox

Although it is hoped that this disease will never be an issue, it certainly deserves mention.

1) Incubation time after exposure to this virus is about 2 weeks. The first symptoms are flulike. When mouth sores and the pox rash develop 3 days later, patients become contagious.
2) Contagiousness is less than for the flu or chicken pox. Several hours of close contact with an infected person usually are needed to transmit the virus. It is spread by droplets in the air.
3) Remaining immunity from vaccinations prior to 1972 is controversial and speculative.
4) New vaccinations will be provided to the military, hospital workers, etc., in case of an attack. Additional vaccine will be used to surround areas where the disease strikes. The vaccine begins working in about 3 days. Vaccination will be voluntary for the population beginning in the year 2004.
5) Side effects from the vaccine can be severe. Fifty out of a million who received the vaccination had a severe complication such as encephalitis (brain inflammation). One person died. The new diluted vaccine may have fewer side effects.
6) A vaccine antidote called vaccinia immune globulin is being prepared and may help with some of the side effects.
7) A new antiviral drug called cidifovir may be useful for the treatment of smallpox.

Smoking Cessation

One out of every 5 deaths in the U.S. results from smoking. A few conditions that are associated with smoking include heart attacks, stroke, lung cancer, osteoporosis, emphysema, pancreatic cancer, leukemia, kidney cancer, breast cancer, pancreatic cancer and many more awful diseases.

The benefits of quitting are enormous. Some examples include extending life an extra 10 years, reducing lung cancer after even 1 year and arresting the development of emphysema. Cessation involves a state of readiness on your part. Quit for yourself and your rate of success will improve. Smoking isn't logical. In fact, according to Dr. C. Everett Koop, nicotine is 10 times more addicting than heroin. Smoking is associated with cues such as being on the phone, riding in the car, drinking at bars, etc. Finally, many people like to use cigarettes as a stress reducer. Any cessation program must address addiction, behavior and stress.

Here is a sample plan to discuss with your health provider:

1) First and above all, make sure you are ready to take action. You don't have to be confident, but you do need to be in action mode. Write the quit date on your calendar.

2) One month before your quit date begin Zyban. This drug will help to reduce craving. It is the same drug as Wellbutrin, a commonly used antidepressant. Begin at 150 mg per day and increase to 150 mg twice daily on day four. The drug takes about 3 to 4 weeks to become fully effective; hence just taper your smoking by 10% during this time frame. The drug may cause anxiety and some weight loss.

3) On your quit day throw out all your cigarettes, lighters, etc.

4) If you smoke 1 pack per day or more, begin with the 21 mg Nicoderm CQ patch. Use it for at least 4 weeks. Taper the patch by 7 mg every 4 weeks until you are off. In some people this process may take longer. The patch may cause skin irritation, so be sure to alternate the locations of the patch on your trunk or arms on a daily basis. For you hard-core addicts, using the nicotine inhaler during "crisis" moments may be useful. Signs of too much nicotine include nausea and dizziness. The nicotine inhaler looks like a small pen. A nicotine cartridge is placed inside of it and the user takes a puff when needed. Each cartridge lasts about 20 minutes. The inhaler may be used instead of the patch or in addition to the patch under your doctor's guidance.

5) Be sure to follow up with your physician 2 weeks after quitting. Remember, nicotine is more addicting than heroin and follow-up by your health care adviser is essential.

6) Continue Zyban for at least 3 months. Often many ex-smokers need to take this medicine for 6 to 12 months.

7) Take each day at a time, rather than dwelling on the whole task. Yesterday's history, tomorrow's a mystery and today is a gift!

8) Be aware of the cues that increase your chances of smoking such as stress, coffee, alcohol, the car, the phone, etc. You may have to change the cue in order to avoid smoking again. For example, you may need to stop drinking alcohol and coffee, if there is a strong association to smoke. You may have to answer the phone in a different room, spray air freshener in your car, and do the dishes immediately after dinner to avoid the cues that cause you to smoke.

9) Decrease stress by quitting at a decent time for you. Consider seeing a psychotherapist with your health provider.

10) Remember to exercise regularly to avoid the weight gain and reduce the stress.
11) Consider using cinnamon sticks and chewing gum as a substitute for smoking.
12) *Please note that 1 cigarette will hurt, and you have come too far to turn back.* Keep these thoughts circulating through your mind. Additionally, the health benefits are enormous. Both the quantity and quality of your life will be enhanced. Even if you relapse, never stop trying. The average smoker may take 3 to 5 times before smoking cessation is achieved. If you learn from past mistakes, you really haven't failed.

Surgical Issues

Remember that vitamins and herbs are drugs and have certain side effects and specific interactions. For instance, ginkgo and Coumadin shouldn't be combined due to increased blood-thinning effects. Be sure to stop ginkgo, valerian, kava kava, St. John's wort and ginseng 2 weeks before surgery to help prevent interactions with anesthesia. Always check with your doctor and pharmacist about herb and vitamin side effects and interactions. Aspirin may need to be stopped 2 weeks before surgery due to bleeding issues. Beta blockers may help to reduce heart complications in patients undergoing noncardiac surgery who have heart disease.

An over-the-counter cream called ELA-Max can be used to numb the pain of blood drawing or IVs. It is a 4% lidocaine cream that is well absorbed into the skin and works in about one-half hour. The cream may be used in kids, too. This drug may be helpful in reducing the discomfort of an IV before surgery.

Spinal anesthesia seems to have fewer side effects such as pneumonia, blood clots, bleeding and even death when compared with general anesthesia.

Also make sure you know what medications to take before surgery. For example, usually it is advisable to take blood pressure medications the morning of surgery and not take oral diabetic medicine. Have your primary care physician perform a physical exam and laboratory evaluation before going to surgery.

West Nile Virus

Okay, who brought this nasty stuff here? Almost every state east of Texas has reported virus activity. I'm sure more states will be reporting increased activity of this virus in the future. Most of the fatalities occur in the elderly. Here are some key features:

1) The first case was isolated in Uganda in 1937.
2) One in 5 develops a mild fever. One in 150 develops meningitis and/or encephalitis (inflammation of the brain).
3) Important clues to this disease include marked muscle weakness and meningitis and/or encephalitis, especially in the late summer months.
4) Advanced age is the biggest risk factor for this ailment.
5) The local or state health department can run an antibody test on the serum or spinal fluid to diagnose this virus.
6) There is no cure for this illness at this time; therefore, prevention is the best and only option.
7) Avoid outdoor activities between dusk and dawn since mosquitoes are most active at this time. The disease may be transmitted via a mosquito bite, blood transfusion, breast feeding and organ donation.
8) Chlorinate your swimming pools. Mosquitoes love water. Don't let water collect in your yard, recycling bin, garbage, pots, empty tires, containers, birdbaths, etc.

9) Deet, a mosquito repellent, is quite effective. Don't apply to infants less than 2 months of age, and use only concentrations of 10% or less on children. A 10 to 50% concentration is adequate for adults. Please read the instructions on the bottle. Deet is currently the best repellent against mosquito bites.

10) About 200 deaths and 4,000 cases of this disease were reported in 2002. New cases have been seen west of the Mississippi. Thousands of cases also may have been unreported due to mild disease.

Chapter Two

Cancer and Early Detection

Cancer is the second-leading cause of death in our nation. Early detection and prevention remain our best defense against this dreaded disease. This chapter covers the latest early-detection techniques and a brief synopsis of the most common cancers.

Bladder Cancer

Smoking, aniline dye exposure, schistosomiasis (a parasite that is often contracted in Africa, the Middle East and the Caribbean) and chronic urinary infection are predisposing factors. Stop smoking and drink several glasses of water daily to prevent this disease. Have a urine analysis performed as a part of a physical examination. Sometimes microscopic blood may be detected. This may be a sign of bladder or kidney cancer.

Breast Cancer

Twelve percent of women will develop breast cancer in their lifetime. Risk factors include obesity, smoking, infertility, uterine cancer, family history and having your first baby past the age of thirty.

Begin mammograms at age 40, repeat every 2 years and continue yearly after age 50. Mammograms pick up 85%

of breast cancers and probably save lives, especially between the ages of 50 and 70. There is debate regarding the efficacy of mammograms between the ages of 40 and 49. The breast self-exam may be useful in detecting lumps, but it hasn't been shown in clinical studies to save lives.

Tamoxifen can help high-risk women cut the chance of breast cancer in half. It is especially effective in women between 40 and 60 years of age who have a family history of breast cancer. A regimen for prevention might include Tamoxifen (in high-risk postmenopausal women), exercise, omega-3 fatty acids (found in salmon and other fish), broccoli (especially broccoli sprouts), soy, green tea and coenzyme Q-10. Don't smoke, and keep alcohol to two drinks or less per day. Evista, a drug similar to Tamoxifen, can reduce breast cancer by 84% but is not FDA-approved for this indication.

How do you know if you are at higher risk for breast cancer? If you answer two or more of the following questions yes and you are 35 or older, check with your doctor because your risk may be higher than normal for breast cancer. Are you over age 60? Has your sister, mother or daughter had breast cancer? Have you ever had a breast biopsy? Did you begin your period before age 12? Did you have your first child after age 30, or are you childless?

Finally, if any first-degree relative has had breast or ovarian cancer before age 50, consider genetic testing for the BRCA-1 and the BRCA-2 gene. About 5 to 10% of breast and ovarian cancer are inherited, and genetic testing in these groups can help intensify screening techniques in your family. Interestingly, Tamoxifen works to help prevent breast cancer in patients with the BRCA-2 gene but not the BRCA-1 gene.

Soy and mistletoe (Iscador) are probably unhelpful for the treatment of breast cancer. Stick with proven therapies.

Cervical Cancer and Pap Smears

The Pap smear is the best screening test ever developed. Obtain this test yearly, or you may obtain it every 2 to 3 years once two Pap smears in a row are normal.

Begin screening at age 18, earlier if you're sexually active. Of the 13,000 women who develop cervical cancer, 50% of them have never had a Pap smear. Human papilloma virus (HPV), smoking, young age at first sexual intercourse and multiple sexual partners are risk factors for cervical cancer.

A screening device for home testing will become available for the early detection of cervical cancer. This test will screen for HPV, which is thought to be the primary cause of this tumor. This test does not replace the pelvic exam done by your physician. During this exam your doctor can feel for pelvic masses and other abnormalities.

If you had a hysterectomy for benign disease, you do not need a repeat smear.

If your Pap test shows atypical squamous cells of unknown significance (ascus), make sure your doctor tests for the human papilloma virus (HPV), especially if you are under 65. If it is positive for this sexually transmitted virus, have a colposcopy (visualization of the cervix with biopsy). This procedure can help to detect an early cancer. Otherwise have a follow-up Pap smear to see if it clears. If you are over 65, your doctor may recommend estrogen cream to see whether it will clear up these atypical squamous cells.

If atypical glandular cells of unknown significance show up (agus), have an immediate colposcopy and biopsy since 30% of these cases have a serious underlying cause such as cancer of the cervix.

Newer screening techniques designed to enhance the Pap smear include computer-assisted screening and liquid-based thin-layer preparations. Each technique may detect suspicious areas of the cervix earlier; however, these early abnormalities often get better with time. The final word on these newer Pap screens is not out yet.

Colon Cancer

This tumor is the third most common cancer after lung and breast. The lifetime risk of developing this cancer is about 6%. A change in the bowel habits or blood in the stool may alert you that a colon tumor is present. Most often no symptoms are apparent. Early detection can save lives.

Begin flexible sigmoidoscopy, an easy test to examine the left side of the colon, at age 50. Repeat in 1 year and then every 5 years thereafter. This test saves lives because it detects polyps (fleshy growths in the colon) before they turn cancerous. More extensive screening such as colonoscopy should be done if there is an early family history of colon cancer, colon polyps, inflammatory bowel disease (ulcerative colitis or Crohn's disease) or symptoms such as a change in the bowel habits, blood in the stool, etc. This test can be done **for** simple screening every 10 years beginning at age 50, instead of flexible sigmoidoscopy.

Colonoscopy is certainly a more thorough test, and the American College of Gastroenterologists favors colonoscopy as the best screening test for this disease. If a single first-degree relative had colon cancer and was over age 60 at the time, screen with colonoscopy at age 40 and repeat every 10 years. If the first-degree relative was less than 60, begin screening in yourself at age 40 and repeat colonoscopy every 3 to 5 years. Recommendations vary considerably, however, and this is but one screening regimen. The United States Preventive Services Task Force (USPSTF) indicates that if a single first-degree relative had colon cancer and was over 60, flexible sigmoidoscopy should begin at age 50 and be done every 5 years. The USPSTF was not convinced that colonoscopy saved lives in such an individual.

Equally important is screening for occult blood in the

stool with the use of stool slides. This should begin at age 50 and be done yearly. This test also has been shown to save lives.

Additional methods for possible prevention of colon cancer include taking an aspirin daily, increasing calcium intake, taking at least 400 mcg of folic acid daily, estrogen, exercise (vigorous exercise at the equivalent of climbing 89 flights of stairs per day reduced colon cancer by 40%) and following the screening procedures described above. Increased fiber intake does not seem to be helpful in reducing this cancer.

The preparation for colonoscopy involves taking Go-Lytely, a large volume of bad-tasting liquid, before the procedure. Try sucking on popsicles between gulps. Another alternative includes Visicol. Take 20 tabs the night before and 20 tabs the morning of the test. Take 3 tabs at a time with a full glass of water. There is less to drink and no bad taste, however electrolyte problems and fluid overload can occur. Don't take Visicol if you have heart, liver or kidney disease. Ginger ale can be taken with Visicol to help prevent a film that sometimes develops on the colon with this preparation. Fleet Phospho-soda is also effective to clean out the colon and requires less fluid intake. Dehydration and kidney failure may occur with this preparation, however, especially in the elderly. Don't take iron or aspirin within 1 week of the procedure. If you are on Coumadin (a blood thinner), let your physician know so the appropriate advice can be given.

Esophageal Carcinoma and Heartburn

This cancer has been rising rapidly since 1975. Predisposing factors include excessive alcohol, smoking and heartburn. Heartburn left untreated at one episode a week can increase the chances of esophageal carcinoma by eightfold. Reduce heartburn by avoiding anti-inflammatories (ibuprofen, aspirin, etc.), alcohol, smoking, fatty foods, caffeine, mints, citrus, chocolate, lying down after a meal and perhaps stress. Prilosec, Prevacid, Nexium, Protonix and Aciphex are excellent medicines to shut down acid production and work very well for heartburn. Esophageal cancer may manifest with swallowing difficulty and weight loss.

Lung Cancer

This is the leading cause of cancer deaths in males and females. It kills more people than cancer of the colon, prostate and breast combined.

Women are more susceptible than men and seem to contract it earlier and with less smoking.

It takes 15 years of smoking cessation to reduce your risk of lung cancer to near normal. More lung cancers are diagnosed in former smokers than current smokers. Other causes include asbestos and radon gas. (Screen your house with a kit from your hardware store.)

Symptoms can include a chronic cough, hoarseness, coughing blood, etc. Consider being screened if you (1) have a personal or strong family history of lung cancer, (2) are older than 40, have smoked a pack per day for 30 years, and have an abnormal result in a breathing test called office spirometry, (3) are exposed to occupational hazards that cause lung cancer such as asbestos, (4) have chronic cough, wheezing and mucous secretion.

The best screening tests include a CAT scan of the chest to detect peripheral lung cancers and sputum cytology to detect central lung cancers that don't show up on CAT scans. (This is done by sending sputum that you cough up to a lab, which looks for abnormal cells under the microscope.) This has worked well in Japan where 5-year survival has increased from 34% to 58%, compared to the USA where 5-year survival remains at a dismal 13%.

Screening is done in Japan where it is hardly done at all in the USA. More studies are required regarding the usage of CAT scans in the early detection of lung cancer.

Early diagnosis is the key to curing this disease. Better yet, never start the deadly habit of smoking. Those of you in high school or college, heed this warning! Nicotine from cigarettes is 10 times more addicting than heroin. Once you're addicted, it is very hard to quit.

Ovarian Cancer

This disease is genetic in 10% and is related to mutations in the tumor-supressor genes BRCA-1 (on chromosone 17) and BRCA-2 (on chromosone 13). About 1 out of 70 women develop this disease. Breast cancer is much more common and develops in 1 out of 9 women.

Risk factors include infertility, family history of breast, ovarian, pancreatic, colon and uterine cancer, obesity, age over 50 and long-term estrogen replacement treatment.

A transvaginal ultrasound takes a few minutes to do and detects ovarian carcinoma at an earlier stage than routine Pap and pelvic exams. Nearly 80% of cancers were found to be in stage 1 via ultrasound versus 55% with routine care. Ca-125, a blood test for ovarian cancer, is controversial. Fibroids, endometriosis, hepatitis and other ailments may raise Ca-125. Many women have normal Ca-125 with early disease. Optimal screening techniques are under study. Perhaps a Ca-125 test combined with transvaginal ultrasound will prove cost-effective in selective individuals.

LPA, or serum lysophosphatadic acid, detected 9 out of 10 patients with stage 1 ovarian cancer. The test missed only 5% of ovarian cancers and was about 90% specific in detecting this disease. Serum proteomic patterns (a special blood test) did not miss any patient with ovarian cancer in a small study. Additionally the test was 95% specific in identifying this disease. Both of these screening tests provide hope for earlier detection of this cancer in the future. These tests should be available soon.

Pancreatic Cancer

This cancer represents the fifth leading cause of cancer death in the USA and has the lowest overall survival at less than 3% at 5 years. Symptoms may include weight loss, abdominal/back pain, itching, weakness and nausea. Risk factors include increased height, diabetes, obesity and smoking. Since there are no effective screening tests for this disease, prevention remains our best option. Physical activity seems to decrease the rate of this deadly disease, especially if you are overweight. An aspirin a day may reduce pancreatic cancer by 43%.

Prostate Cancer

This tumor accounts for 10% of all male cancer deaths. Risk is increased 8 times if a first—or second-degree relative has it. Symptoms can include blood in the urine, urinary obstruction, bone pain, etc.

Help to prevent this tumor by increasing lycopene (an ingredient found in tomatoes that seemed to reduce prostate cancer in a Harvard study), and by taking vitamin E at a dose of 400 units a day. Vitamin E reduced the number of aggressive prostate tumors. Actually, dosages as low as 50 units per day were useful in preventing early prostate tumors from becoming more advanced.

Lycopene, given to patients with prostate cancer who are awaiting surgery, reduced the tumor grade (aggressiveness of the tumor). A dose of 15 mg twice daily was given 3 weeks before surgery. Lycopene seems to shrink prostate tumors and lower PSAs.

Also 2 servings of fatty fish per week may help to reduce

prostate cancer in half, compared to people who didn't consume fish at all.

Proscar, which reduces prostate size, is presently being studied for the prevention of prostate cancer.

Obtain an annual rectal exam and blood test called a PSA beginning at age 50. Begin at age 40 if there is a family history of prostate cancer or if you are African American. Please note that 25% of patients with prostate cancer have a normal PSA; hence it isn't a perfect screening test.

We're still not sure whether the PSA test saves lives; however, I suspect that it will eventually be proven. Up to 80% of prostate cancers are diagnosed confined to the prostate, whereas before PSA screening occurred, only 30% of prostate tumors were localized in the prostate. (Before PSA screening most tumors had spread outside of the prostate.) An Austrian study showed a 42% reduction in mortality after 5 years for men having PSA screening versus the men who received no screening.

Generally, a PSA is normal if it is between 0 and 4. Higher levels may reflect benign enlargement, a prostate infection, or prostate cancer. If the PSA is normal but increasing rapidly, for example, more than 0.75 point per year, this may be a sign of prostate cancer even though the PSA is still normal. Finally, the PSA must be adjusted according to your age. For Caucasians in their 40s, for example, the PSA is abnormal if it is over 2.5.

An herb, pc-spes, is a combination of saw palmetto and Chinese herbs. This herb has fallen out of favor for the treatment of this disease. Surgery still offers the best chance at cure and is better than radiation or observation alone.

Skin Cancer

Sunburn is a risk factor for melanoma (a malignant skin cancer). Wear sunscreen lotion that blocks ultraviolet rays (UVA and UVB) with an SPF of at least 15. Wind, heat, altitude and humidity (including exposure to water) can decrease the effectiveness of sunscreens. An SPF over 35 only increases the cost and **does**n't offer much more protection. Apply sunscreen liberally to the skin 20 minutes before sunbathing and then every 2 hours thereafter. Also reapply after swimming.

Early detection can be accomplished by doing a routine skin exam yearly. Use a hand mirror to look at the nape of the neck, the soles of the feet, the back of the legs, etc. A recent change in a mole is often the earliest sign of skin cancer. Also look for irregular borders and multiple colors while examining your moles. These signs might also signal skin cancer.

Can skin cancer be prevented? At this time sunscreens may reduce DNA damage and actinic keratoses (forerunners of skin cancer). We do not know whether they will reduce the incidence of skin cancer. Moderate sun exposure is key.

Chapter Three

Deadly Problems

Accidents and drugs account for many needless deaths in the USA. Here are the keys to help prevent these tragedies.

Automobiles, Boats and Protective Devices

My advice is to buy a car that has air bags and traction control. This should be standard equipment on most cars. Stay even healthier and buy a car with a good safety record (check with *Consumer Reports*).

Check your tire pressure monthly with your own gauge. Keep the tires inflated according to your car's specifications. Mildly low pressure can cause tread separation. Get your brakes checked if you hear a squeaking, grinding noise or if the brake light on the dashboard stays lit. Air bags have saved thousands of lives but there have been a few deaths. Make sure that you are situated at least 10 inches from your steering wheel. Tilt the steering wheel downward so that the air bag points toward your chest and not your face.

Alcohol, speeding and sleep apnea are three common causes of car accidents. Distraction from cell phones, eating, putting on makeup and changing CDs causes about 25% of motor vehicle accidents. Remember to wear your seat belts in the front and the back seats. People do go through the front windshield from the back seat of the car. Such human projectiles can in turn injure or kill the person in the front seat. Do not flip the shoulder belt behind you, because the device will not be as protective. Seat belts reduce death by 65% and air bags add an additional 3%. In addition, the high risk of traffic accidents between the ages of 16 and 24 is attributed to speeding, cell phones, inexperience, drugs and additional people in the car (distraction).

Don't pump antilock brakes as the car may flip over in wet conditions. Just push the brakes down to the floor. The jerking motion and grinding sounds are natural for these brakes. The headrest should make contact just above your ears, to help prevent whiplash injuries.

Wear life preservers on canoes and small boats since rain, other boats, and even a gust of wind can turn a happy time into a catastrophe. Also a sober driver on a boat does not guarantee your safety if you are a passenger: Many boating accidents occur when drunk passengers fall overboard.

Whether it's bicycling, riding a motorcycle or roller-blading, helmets save lives. Remember to wear wrist, elbow, and knee guards while roller-blading.

Bioterrorism

September 11 will never be forgotten. Terrorism is designed to scare the lives of many by threatening the lives of a few.

Let's put this in perspective. A murder probably occurs every minute, and the flu kills more than 20,000 people yearly. Motor vehicle accidents, suicides and smoking wipe out hundreds of thousands of people in the USA every year. We don't think of dying when we get in a car, cross the street or eat high-cholesterol meals. Nuclear bombs and biological warfare, however, are another story.

It is extremely difficult to kill mass numbers of people with biologic weapons. Sure, smallpox, anthrax, plague, botulism and tularemia can kill people, but growing, storing, and disseminating such bacteria is an enormous task. Instead we are growing vaccines, storing antibiotics, and disseminating information to counter this threat. Building, transporting and detonating a nuclear bomb is no simple matter either.

While we should be alert, consider reexamining your beliefs regarding bioterrorism. Remember, when we fear death more than life, we cease to live. Life is sacred whether one dies from the flu, suicide or a terrorist act. Life is about beliefs, and the terrorists have projected the image that millions can be extinguished through biowarfare. If you don't have evidence for this belief, perhaps you have let the terrorists form these beliefs for you. When emotion takes priority over logic, faulty belief systems may develop. Terrorists thrive on faulty beliefs.

Here is an interesting example about faulty beliefs. Consider your beliefs regarding two presidential candidates: The first one drinks excessive alcohol, has illicit affairs and other problems. The second candidate is a patriot and decorated war hero who has an occasional beer and no illicit affairs. Who would get your vote? The first candidate is FDR (Franklin D. Roosevelt), and the second one is Adolph Hitler.

Delve into your own beliefs. Does your belief have any credible evidence? Is the belief really yours or did it come from someone else? Perhaps it came from a friend, a parent or maybe even a terrorist. Take a good hard look!

Bullying

Thirty percent of sixth—to tenth-graders are involved in bullying. This is a form of harassment. Both the bullied and the person doing the bullying are likely having problems with psychosocial adjustment. While this problem is quite prevalent, there are very few proposed solutions on the table.

The following suggestions might be considered in sequence: (1) let the bullied student try to resolve the situation over a finite period of time; (2) consider having a student/teacher board resolve the problem; (3) involve the parents on both sides if necessary; (4) have your attorney write a letter to the parents threatening a lawsuit if the bullying continues. It is important to stop bullying before psychological or physical harm occurs. Victims of bullying often become depressed later in life. Often bullies will become future criminals. Trained student mediators provide the best means to prevent and resolve these conflicts. Encourage your school to initiate a policy to address this very important subject.

Carbon Monoxide

This gas is colorless and odorless. It is produced when fuel is burned. The gas binds to our blood cells and does not allow oxygen to get to our tissues. This can result in severe lung damage, brain damage and even death. While the rates are decreasing due to regulated car emissions, it still remains a major health threat.

Common symptoms include dizziness, headaches, breathing difficulty, confusion, nausea and fainting. If these symptoms occur in an enclosed area, get some fresh air and go to the emergency room. Increased concentrations of oxygen are central to the treatment of this ailment.

Tips for prevention include the following.

1) Buy smoke detectors and carbon monoxide detectors for your home. Place these detectors on each floor. Place the carbon monoxide detectors at least 6 feet from a gas-burning appliance; otherwise the alarm may sound unnecessarily. Make sure you know the expiration date

of your monitor. The alarm tester may still work but the monitor may no longer be able to detect carbon monoxide.

2) Never let a car idle in the garage.
3) Never heat your home with an oven.
4) Don't run fuel-burning equipment such as grills, engines, etc., in an enclosed area.
5) Have your fuel-burning appliances inspected yearly. This may include gas or oil-burning ovens, furnaces, water heaters, etc.
6) Have your chimney and flues inspected yearly.

Dating Violence

One in 5 female students has reported being sexually or physically abused by a dating partner. The risk factors for dating violence include substance abuse, eating disorders, sexual intercourse beginning under age 15, pregnancy, and former suicide attempts in the adolescent female. Counsel your kids early.

Handguns

Purchasing handguns can result in a higher incidence of suicide within a week after purchase and persists up to 6 years. Other studies show that homicides increase as well. The most common reason why 17.5% of the population owns handguns is self-defense, but as you can see the price you pay may be with your own life.

Lightning

Prevention is your best bet because lightning often causes the heart to stop beating. Additionally significant neurological damage can ensue if one survives. If you hear frequent, loud thunder, seek shelter immediately. Also if there is a time gap of less than 30 seconds between the lightning flash and the thunder boom, seek shelter. Every 5-second gap is equivalent to a storm distance of 1 mile. If you are in an open field, kneel with your head low to the ground. It is best to seek shelter in a large building or fully enclosed metal vehicle. If you are in the car, don't touch anything metal. If you are in a building, avoid electrical outlets, electrical cords, telephones, showers, sinks, plumbing fixtures, TV, electrical devices and computers. It is conceivable that lightning could be conducted through these devices.

Smoke Detectors

Place one on each floor so you are alerted in plenty of time. Smoke inhalation and carbon-monoxide poisoning will kill you before the flames do.

Street Drugs

1) Methylenedioxymethamphetamine (ecstasy). This is an amphetamine and can cause hallucinations, anxiety, depression, and paranoia (lasting for weeks). Heart rate and pressure can also increase.
2) Flunitrazepam (roofies). This is the date-rape drug and can result in amnesia and sedation. Always be in possession of your drink. If you put it down, don't pick it up again.
3) Ketamine (special k). This agent can cause chest pain, palpitations, amnesia, euphoria, flashbacks and sedation.
4) GHB (liquid ecstacy). It might build muscles at the expense of your life. It also can cause disinhibition and euphoria and can lead to date rape. Date-rape drugs can be difficult to measure in the urine. A young

woman who suffers from amnesia and sedation may have ingested such a drug.

5) Marijuana. This drug might be linked to respiratory cancers, decreased intelligence, drug dependency and other illicit drug use.

6) Cocaine. It is very addicting and can lead to seizures, nasal septum perforation, asthma, heart attacks and rhythm disturbances. Combined group and individual therapy can be helpful.

7) The bottom line is that drug education needs to take place not only in the schools but also in the home. Talk to your teens about the above dangers of drugs. Show them that you mean business by purchasing a few drug-screening kits through your local pharmacy. The kits can screen for marijuana, cocaine, amphetamines, etc. Tell them that you reserve the right to test them at any time and they may also do the same with you. Now your teens know that you mean business. Additionally you will also serve as an excellent role model. Also emphasize to your child that once he or she sets a beverage down at a party, it should not be picked up again. Slipping drugs into a beverage happens frequently.

Chapter Four

Heart Disease and Early Detection

Heart disease remains the number one killer in the USA. Cholesterol control, smoking cessation, blood pressure monitoring, exercise, medicines and early detection will continue to cut the incidence of this disease.

Aspirin

Certainly if you have had a heart attack or stroke, you are probably on aspirin. This old medicine made from tree bark in 1850 is indeed a wonder drug.

Aspirin is beneficial for preventing heart attacks if you are a man over 40 or a woman past menopause and have two or more of the following risk factors: obesity (30% or more over ideal body weight), high cholesterol, smoking, high blood pressure and early heart disease in your family.

A baby aspirin (81 mg) could help reduce a heart attack by 28% over the next five years! Additional possible benefits may include the prevention of certain cancers, colon polyps and Alzheimer's disease.

The downside of taking aspirin includes silent intestinal bleeding, interactions with Coumadin and aggravation of asthma.

Enteric-coated aspirin does not reduce intestinal bleeding, so take the cheapest baby aspirin with food. Of course, always obtain your doctor's approval first. If you ever develop symptoms of a heart attack, such as chest pain, be sure to chew the aspirin as it will get into your system much faster. If you are having a stroke, don't take an aspirin until a brain scan is done to rule out a bleed in the brain. If a hemorrhage in the brain caused the stroke, aspirin may make the bleeding worse. As indicated, aspirin is very useful to prevent a stroke from occurring.

Cholesterol

High cholesterol may lead to heart disease, stroke, peripheral artery disease, kidney ailments and erectile dysfunction.

Reduce LDL, or bad cholesterol, by quitting smoking, eating Cheerios or oatmeal, taking Metamucil, eating soy (tofu, soy powder, soy milk), eating citrus, exercising, consuming garlic or olive oil and taking Benecol.

Take Control and Benecol are over-the-counter spreads that reduce cholesterol by 10% with very little absorption. The LDL, or bad cholesterol, can be reduced by 15%. Benecol also comes in softgel form, and this preparation reduces cholesterol as well as the spread. The price, however, is considerably higher.

Prescription-medication options for lowering cholesterol include the statin agents, such as Lipitor, Pravachol, Zocor, Mevacor and Lescol XL. These agents are the most effective drugs in lowering the total and LDL cholesterol. Reductions of 30 to 50% can be obtained in the LDL cholesterol and 5 to 10% elevations can be obtained in the HDL, or good cholesterol. Statin agents are excellent drugs to lower heart attacks, strokes and possibly dementia. Additionally, statin medications may reduce the incidence of macular degeneration, kidney disease, osteoporosis and possibly multiple sclerosis. More studies will be forthcoming.

Liver enzymes should be monitored periodically when

one is taking a statin drug, although these drugs rarely cause liver problems. The CPK, a blood test for muscle, should be monitored occasionally as well. If you develop muscle aches on these agents (somewhat common), you should stop the medicine and call your doctor.

Welchol can lower cholesterol by 9 to 18% (3 to 6 pills once daily). It works by binding cholesterol in the gut. Zetia is taken once daily and can reduce the LDL cholesterol an extra 25% when combined with a statin drug. This agent can also mildly raise HDL and lower triglycerides. Gemfibrozil, niacin, and Tricor are most effective at lowering triglycerides (fats) and raising HDL. Dilantin, an antiseizure medicine, raises HDL 50% but has some significant side effects. Gugulipid, an herb that has been used in India since 600 B.C., lowers LDL cholesterol and triglycerides by 10 to 15%. It also lowers HDL by 10%, which may not be good. This herb is undergoing testing in the USA. Red yeast rice products can lower cholesterol like statin drugs and may be obtained at vitamin stores. The side effects are similar to those of the statin agents.

Aim for an LDL below 130, and keep it below 100 if you have known diabetes or heart disease. Keep your HDL or good cholesterol as high as possible (50 or over in women and 45 or over in men). Another good indicator that correlates highly with heart attack risk is the ratio of the total cholesterol to HDL. In other words, if the total cholesterol divided by your HDL is greater than 4, there is a higher incidence of heart attacks. Every 1% one lowers cholesterol decreases heart disease by 2%. Additionally, cholesterol reduction lowers stroke risk by 30%.

Twenty-five percent of heart attacks occur with cholesterol values under 200. Other blood markers that can possibly predict heart disease include CRP, lipoprotein (a), homocysteine and fibrinogen. These may be tested to better define future heart disease in a puzzling individual. For example, if a person has a heart attack without any cardiac risk factors, the above blood tests should be considered. The high-sensitivity CRP (C-reactive protein) and the total cholesterol divided by the HDL remain the best predictors of future heart attacks.

EBCT (electron beam computed tomography) is an X ray that can show plaque in the coronary arteries. It is simply another risk factor for heart disease just as is cholesterol. Consider this expensive, 5-minute test if you are not motivated to prevent heart disease in yourself. The test is not very helpful if you are over 70 or under 35 years of age.

Raise HDL or good cholesterol by losing weight, quitting smoking, and exercising. Also remember to keep fats or triglycerides under 150 since higher fats can lead to increased rates of heart disease. In men who have coronary artery disease, raising HDL by 25% can reduce heart attacks by 25%. The lifestyle trial by Dean Ornish, M.D., demonstrated that coronary disease can be reversed with a low-fat diet, exercise and behavior modification.

Coronary Artery Disease

This is the number one killer in the USA. Risk factors include cigarette smoking, diabetes, hypertension (pressure over 140/90 or on an antihypertensive medicine), HDL (good cholesterol) under 40, family history of early heart disease (male first-degree relative under 55 or female first-degree relative under 65) and your own age (a man 45 or older or a woman 55 or older). Other possible risk factors include a diagonal earlobe crease, baldness in short men, and a high ratio of the length of the index finger to the length of the ring finger on the right hand. (This ratio is predictive of a man's having a heart attack under age 55. The ratio is a negative factor if it is over 1. Measure from the crease closest to the palm.)

Reduce your risk by eating healthy foods, especially

fruits, vegetables, whole-grain foods, nuts (walnuts, peanuts), fish, shellfish, olive oil, etc. High-fiber ingestion in a Finnish study showed a 27% lower risk of coronary death rate. (Much of the fiber consisted of rye bread. Soluble fibers such as oats were also protective). Consider taking a coated aspirin a day (may reduce stroke and reduces heart attacks by 20%). Aerobic exercise 3 to 4 times a week can reduce heart attacks by 30 to 40%.

Taking at least 400 mcg of folic acid (B12 and B6 are also useful) can reduce homocysteine, a chemical that clogs arteries in our heart and brain. Additionally, B vitamins have been found to reduce restenosis after angioplasty (lesser blockages in a vessel after it is opened). Q-Gel, a unique brand of coenzyme Q-10, helps to prevent the bad cholesterol (LDL) from sticking to our arteries. It also helps to increase the pumping power of our hearts and has protected mammals against strokes. (See www. DrLipkis.com) Vitamin E decreases nonfatal heart attacks by 50%, according to a Cambridge study involving more than 19,000 patients. Other studies, however, show no reduction in heart mortality with vitamin E. A recent study showed that green tea can reduce the incidence of heart attacks by 50%. Remember to brew it, and don't add milk to the tea because that binds the antioxidants. Green tea thins the blood and helps to prevent the bad cholesterol from sticking to our arteries. Green tea capsules are easier to consume and are available at the above website. One to two cups of green tea per day probably has a cardioprotective effect. Ten cups per day may help to prevent cancer. Finally, one or two glasses of wine a day can reduce coronary artery disease and decrease cancer incidence. If you have a personal or family history of alcoholism, however, don't drink at all.

Also remember to keep your sugar below 110, your blood pressure below 140/90, your LDL (bad cholesterol) below 130 (below 100 if you have coronary disease or diabetes), your triglycerides (fats) below 150, your HDL (good cholesterol) above 45 if male and above 50 if female, your body mass index below 27 (see Appendix B) and don't smoke at all (including cigarettes, cigars, chewing tobacco, etc.). Playing the "numbers game" is very important to help prevent heart attacks.

Fish oil also can help prevent coronary disease. Try one or two servings of fish per week. According to Dr. Dean Ornish, a low-fat diet (10% fat), stress reduction, walking 3 times per week, smoking cessation and group support can reverse coronary blockages and reduce coronary events. The study included only 48 patients but is still impressive.

An ACE inhibitor, such as Altace, can reduce the incidence of heart attacks, strokes and new-onset diabetes (according to the HOPE trial). Pravachol can help lower the incidence of first-time heart attacks by one-third in men and women with high cholesterol (West of Scotland study). This drug also reduced the incidence of coronary disease in high-risk elderly patients (Prosper study). Zocor reduced heart attacks and strokes in patients with heart disease risk factors even without elevated cholesterol. Patients with low bad cholesterol (LDL less than 116) benefited from the use of this drug, according to the Heart Protection trial. Niacin, when combined with Zocor, reduced coronary events by 90% in patients who had a history of coronary heart disease. Niaspan is the best-tolerated sustained-release niacin. Potassium can help to decrease blood pressure and strokes. At least 5 servings of fruits and vegetables daily can supply adequate potassium. Finally, if you have coronary artery disease, keep the LDL below 100, and raise the HDL. Screen for coronary disease by obtaining a CRP (see later in this chapter) or obtaining a heart scan.

Heart CT scans may detect coronary disease earlier by finding calcium deposits in the cholesterol plaque. Such plaque is likely stable as it has calcified and is unlikely to rupture. The dangerous plaque is probably the noncalcified plaque, which is more likely to crack open, bleed and cause a heart attack. Heart scans are unable to detect this. A CRP test can be helpful in detecting unstable plaque. What about stress tests? Most people (68%) who have heart attacks have less than 50% plaque in their coronary arteries. Stress tests detect blockages that are 75% or more, hence this test is an ineffective screen. Heart attacks occur when this plaque cracks or ruptures. Blood clots around the obstruction and blood flow to the heart muscle ceases, resulting in the attack. While a stress test cannot screen for early obstructions in the coronary arteries, it can predict future cardiac risk in another way. After peak exercise on the stress test, the heart rate should fall about 15 to 25 beats per minute once a person stops exercising. If your heart rate falls at less than 12 beats per minute, there is a greater future mortality (20% versus 5% over the next 6 years).

CPR

When a person's heart stops, the individual becomes unconscious and will die unless the heart is revived and oxygenated bleed gets to the brain. The recommendations indicate to perform chest compressions without checking for the pulse. The delay in finding and verifying a pulse is just too long. Give 100 chest compressions in a minute if the person is 8 years or older. It is acceptable to do chest compressions without ventilation (mouth-to-mouth) if the rescuer is unwilling to perform this task due to fear of infection or difficulty in doing this procedure. One study showed that chest compressions alone were just as useful as chest compression and mouth-to-mouth.

Honor do-not-resuscitate orders if made clear by immediate family members. Family members should be allowed to attend resuscitation measures, depending on the situation. These may be the last moments of a person's life.

CRP

This is an interesting blood test that measures for inflammation in the arteries. Specifically, the test is for high-sensitivity C-reactive protein, or hs-CRP.

Atherosclerosis begins as an inflammatory reaction in the vessel wall. This test is better than a cholesterol panel at predicting your chances of having a stroke and heart attack. It is an inexpensive blood test. Inflammatory factors released by coronary plaque causes the liver to release CRP, which is a strong predictor of heart disease, even 7 years ahead of time! The Framingham study shows that men or women in the highest quartile for CRP and systolic blood pressure double their stroke risk.

Statin drugs, which are used to lower cholesterol, can lower this risk factor for coronary disease and stroke. Niacin, mild alcohol consumption (1–2 drinks per day) and Evista (a drug for osteoporosis) also lower CRP.

Besides the CRP, the total cholesterol divided by the HDL, or good cholesterol, is an excellent indicator of heart disease. Aim for a ratio of less than 4. Higher values correlate with more frequent cardiac events. Even if you have a normal LDL, or bad cholesterol, the CRP can be elevated and be predictive of a future cardiac event.

Fat Clarification

You need fats to live, but some are better than others. Saturated fats include fatty meats, high-fat dairy products and certain oils (palm and coconut). These fats raise cholesterol and the bad, or LDL, cholesterol. Trans fatty acids are equally bad and are found in stick margarines, high-fat milk, butter, cheese and commercially processed baked goods (often contain "partially hydrogenated" on the label). Trans fats also raise LDL cholesterol and may be responsible for 30,000 deaths per year. Soft-tub margarine and Benecol spread are fine to use.

Polyunsaturated fats such as corn, safflower, sunflower and cottonseed oil lower the LDL, or bad cholesterol, and lower HDL, or good cholesterol. We still like to restrict these oils as we do not know the effects they have on heart disease.

Monounsaturated fats include almonds, olive oil, peanut oil, canola oil, macadamia nuts, walnuts and pistachio nuts. These fats lower LDL and keep the HDL steady. These fats are considered to be healthy. Nuts can lower the incidence of sudden death due to coronary disease and even type 2 diabetes! Think about replacing high-calorie snacks with a tablespoon of peanut butter or an ounce of nuts daily.

Omega-3 fat, a type of polyunsaturated and monounsaturated fat, is healthy since it lowers cholesterol and triglycerides and probably the incidence of heart disease. Omega-3 fats include fish oil, canola oil, macadamia nuts and oil, flaxseed oil and soybean oil. It appears that fish oil, canola oil and macadamia nuts or oil top the list for the healthiest fats.

Fish

A weekly serving of fish can reduce heart attacks by 40% and can reduce sudden death. Fish oil consists of two main ingredients, EPA (eicosapentaenoic acid) and DHA (docosahexaenoic acid). These healthy oils are especially found in salmon, mackerel and herring. These fish oils are probably the ingredients in fish that help to prevent heart attacks. Even shellfish contains some omega fatty acids.

An Italian study shows that among 11,000 heart attack survivors, fish oil (875 mg of omega fatty acids daily) reduced the incidence of fatal and nonfatal heart attacks and strokes. There was a 45% reduction in heart attacks over three and one-half years. Fish oil also may help to slow the progression of chronic kidney failure.

The omega-3 fish oils (EPA and DHA) also may help to improve memory, depression, manic-depressive illness, autoimmune disorders (such as rheumatoid arthritis and inflammatory bowel disease), cholesterol and triglycerides. Two servings of fish per week may help to prevent prostate cancer.

Try fish oil capsules if you don't like fish, and take two 1,000 mg capsules of fish oil daily. Each 1-gram capsule of fish oil usually contains 300 mg of omega-3 fatty acids, which consist of DHA and EPA (both are omega-3 fatty acids). Consider an extra-strength brand, which contains 840 mg of omega-3 fatty acids. (The DHA and EPA omega-3 fatty acids add up to 840 mg.)

Heart Failure

This is the number one cause of hospitalization in the elderly in the USA. The main cause of congestive heart failure is coronary artery disease; other causes include hypertension, heart valve disorders and cardiomyopathy (muscle problem within the heart). Obesity may also contribute to heart failure.

Major symptoms include needing to rest on a few pillows at night, waking up at night feeling short of breath, crackles in the lungs on exam, an extra heart sound on exam, distended neck veins on exam and a large heart on chest X ray. Minor symptoms include leg swelling, nocturnal cough, a large liver and a pleural effusion (fluid in the lung). The diagnosis is made with two major criteria or one major and two minor criteria. Generally if there is shortness of breath, fatigue, cough and leg swelling, consider heart failure as a cause.

A simple and inexpensive blood test that measures a

hormone called BNP (B natriuretic peptide) is 95% accurate in both diagnosing heart failure and excluding it.

ACE inhibitor medicines (Altace, Zestril, Accupril, for example) can decrease mortality by 50 to 73%. The diuretic spironolactone can reduce death rate by 30% in severe heart failure. Beta blockers (Coreg, Toprol XL) can also reduce heart-failure mortality by one-third. Exercise training, diuretics and a low-cholesterol, low-salt diet can be beneficial. Coenzyme Q-10, an antioxidant, may also be helpful. Digoxin, Inocor, Natrecor and Dobutamine help the heart pump stronger but don't decrease mortality. These agents may reduce hospitalizations. Cardiac resynchronization therapy (CRT) is a special pacemaker that allows both ventricles (the pumping chambers of the heart) to pump at the same time. In other words, in selected patients this device helps the heart pump more efficiently. Sometimes automatic implantable carioverter defibrillators (AICD) are placed in the heart to avoid fatal heart-rhythm disturbances. This device is especially helpful in heart-failure patients who have had a recent heart attack. It is also helpful if the heart failure has caused a rhythm disturbance called sustained ventricular tachycardia. This heart-rhythm problem can be fatal, and the AICD saves lives by shocking the heart out of this bad rhythm.

If a test such as echocardiogram (which looks at the heart-pumping ability) or a BNP is abnormal, an ACE inhibitor and a beta blocker should be considered. These medicines should be added even if there are no symptoms yet the above tests are abnormal. Sometimes an ACE inhibitor will cause patients to cough, and the medication needs to be discontinued. In this case an ARB may be tried. This class of drugs, also effective in treating heart failure, includes Cozaar, Diovan, Atacand, Avapro, etc. Finally, your weight should be monitored meticulously. If there is an abrupt change in your weight, your nurse practitioner, physician assistant or physician should be contacted immediately. For example, if you gain 3 pounds quickly, then the dosage of your diuretic may need to be increased.

Also consider a sleep study. Airway obstruction during sleep may be a sign of sleep apnea. This condition may aggravate heart failure and is treatable with CPAP, or continuous, positive airway pressure. In other words, you wear a mask that allows pressurized air to keep the airway open.

Mediterranean Diet

This outstanding diet contains fruits, vegetables, seeds, nuts, olive oil, beans and fish. Wine is consumed as well (recommend no more than 1 to 2 glasses a day). This diet, which comes from southern Italy, Greece and Crete, seems to be associated with long life spans, reduced heart disease and reduced cancers.

A 36% increased survival is seen with cancer patients on a Mediterranean diet. Another study showed a significant reduction in heart attacks and total mortality in patients with heart disease who followed a Mediterranean diet (the Lyon study).

Metabolic Syndrome and Heart Disease Risk

This syndrome is of particular importance because if you have it, your risk for developing heart disease and diabetes goes up. Criteria for this syndrome include 3 or more of the following: abdominal obesity (a waist circumference of over 102 cm in men and over 88 cm in women), high triglycerides or fats in the blood (over 150), low HDL, or good cholesterol (under 40 in men and under 50 in women), high blood pressure (130/85 or above) and an elevated fasting blood sugar (110 or above). Nearly 25% of the nation has this syndrome. Dietary education and exercise remain the cornerstone of treatment. The use of

Niaspan (niacin) may help to raise HDL and lower triglycerides. It is hoped that lifestyle and drug treatment of this newly recognized syndrome will help reduce the risk for heart disease.

Stroke

A stroke is essentially a brain attack. It is the third-leading cause of death in the United States. In most cases there is inadequate blood flow to the brain and a section of it ceases to function. This may result in speech problems, walking difficulties, weakness, numbness and other such neurological symptoms.

A stroke may occur as a result of cholesterol plaque being thrown from the heart or nearby vessels. It may also occur secondary to a hemorrhage in the brain or a blockage in a vessel that directly feeds nutrients to the brain. There are many ways to prevent a stroke. Here are a few key items.

1) Controlling blood pressure can reduce initial strokes by 40%. Keep the pressure at least under 140/90. If you have had previous vascular disease, maintain the pressure under 130/85. Blood pressure control can also reduce the chance of a second stroke after an initial one has occurred. Thiazide diuretics and ACE inhibitors are the best antihypertensive drugs to lower stroke risk.

2) Pravachol and Zocor can reduce the chance of a first stroke by one-third due to their cholesterol-lowering effects.

3) Aspirin thins the blood and can be very effective in preventing a stroke after a first one has occurred. If a stroke is in progress, don't take an aspirin until a hemorrhage in the brain is first ruled out with a brain scan. Since aspirin thins the blood, it may aggravate a hemorrhagic-type stroke. Aspirin probably does not

prevent a first stroke from occurring if one has no symptoms.

4) ACE inhibitors such as Altace and Aceon (when combined with a diuretic) can help to prevent a stroke. Both of these agents lower blood pressure. The stroke-reducing effect, however, exceeds what can be expected from blood-pressure lowering alone. Altace works best before a first stroke occurs, especially if there is associated heart disease. Aceon in combination with a diuretic works best in preventing future strokes after one has occurred.

5) Adding 1 to 2 servings a day of a potassium-rich food such as orange juice or bananas can reduce the number of strokes by 40%. Another food that has a stroke-reducing effect is fiber.

6) Smoking cessation can reduce strokes by 50% after the first 2 years. This has been seen in observational trials. At this time, blood pressure control is more important for the prevention of stroke than smoking cessation.

7) Keeping your blood sugar controlled is helpful in preventing kidney, eye and nerve problems in diabetics (small vessel problems). At the present time, controlling sugar does not prevent strokes, which occurs mainly in the large vessels.

8) Raising HDL, or good cholesterol, can also decrease the incidence of strokes. Exercise, weight loss, smoking cessation and certain drugs (statins, niacin and fibrates) can raise HDL and therefore cut down the incidence of this deadly disease.

9) Aggrenox, Ticlid and Plavix are blood thinners that can help to prevent secondary strokes after a first one has occurred. These agents are modestly better than aspirin but much more costly. Coumadin, another blood thinner, helps to prevent strokes as a result of atrial fibrillation. This is a rhythm disorder of the heart that results in

cholesterol plaque being thrown from the heart to the brain.

10) Surgical correction of carotid-artery blockages may be helpful after a transient stroke or mild stroke has occurred. The carotid arteries feed the brain their blood supply from the neck. This surgery works best when there is a 70 to 99% carotid blockage in a patient who has symptoms of a recent transient stroke. A transient stroke may manifest as temporary speech difficulties, blindness in an eye, weakness in a limb, etc. Often this temporary stroke or transient ischemic attack will last from 15 to 30 minutes. It is controversial whether such surgery is helpful in preventing a first stroke when there is a 70 to 99% blockage and no associated symptoms. These studies are applicable if your vascular surgeon has less than a 6% complication rate for this surgery.

Chapter Five

Helpful Hints

Sometimes the little things that we do can have an enormous impact on our lives. Harness this power by following the helpful hints below.

Learning

Keep your mind sharp, and never lose your desire to learn new ideas. My promise to you is that I will continually update this longevity book to reflect the latest information. You can only benefit from this handbook by reading and rereading the valuable information contained within. Promise me you will do that! Remember, the brain is a muscle and must be exercised.

Medic Alert Band, Bracelet or Necklace

Call 1-800-432-5378 and obtain an engraved necklace that lists, for example, your allergies or major medical conditions. An ID number on the jewelry allows the paramedic or ER doctor to call to obtain a comprehensive list of your medicines, allergies and medical conditions.

Medic Alert is the name of the nonprofit company, and confidentiality is guaranteed. Approximate cost is $35 for the first year and $15 yearly. Update your records anytime. This is a lifesaver.

Get help at home. If you are prone to falls due to arthritis, heart disease, diabetes, neurological diseases, etc., obtain an alert device that can go around your neck. If you are hurt, you can push a button that will alert a monitoring station. The police can subsequently be notified by the staff that you are hurt. This device will work while you are in the house. Call AARP at 1-800-424-3410 to see what current vendors they recommend.

Medications

Always get a written description from your pharmacist for any medication, vitamin or herb that you take. This description should include all side effects and interactions.

If you start or change a medication, let your physician know. Please do not stop a medication without first telling your physician. So many people stop their medicines because of excessive cost, too many pills, a minor side effect or lack of perceived benefit.

For example, a cholesterol-lowering medicine may cost a lot and cause mild muscle aches in Mr. Jones. Additionally, Mr. Jones doesn't feel any better on the medicine. If he had called his physician, the doctor might have said, "Mr. Jones, did you know that you are cutting your risk for stroke and heart attack by 33%? The mild muscle aches may be a side effect of the medication. Stop the medicine temporarily today and come in for a simple blood test. I anticipate that we will be able to restart this life-saving drug shortly." Communicate your beliefs to your doctor. You may be having some misconceptions that could threaten your well-being. Let your doctor have some input.

Poison Alert

I am happy to say that we now have a national poison hotline! The number is 1-800-222-1222. This number can be used anywhere in the USA to obtain urgent poison information.

Many poisonings occur daily, so call the poison hotline and obtain "Poison Help" stickers and magnets. This will prove especially useful for parents and grandparents. Emergency rooms are not always prepared to handle these types of calls due to patient volume. Keep this number handy.

Religion

The universe seems too orderly to me for it to be a fluke. Having some sort of belief system helps to give our life meaning, hope and order. Additionally, there are studies to imply that religion helps to increase interleukins, chemicals that augment our immune systems.

Prayer also can help to reduce complications and mortality in an intensive-care unit setting. In one particular hospital study, the patients who had a better outcome did not even know that others were praying for them for a total of 4 weeks!

Of course, religion is an area that you may not be able to measure scientifically. Certainly your beliefs are entirely up to you.

Test Results

Make sure that you always ask for a verbal or written result of any test that you have. This is a common mistake made by patients throughout the country. "I didn't hear from the doctor so everything must be fine." Never assume that no news is good news. Call your physician if you don't receive your results in a timely manner. Keep all your lab results and medical papers in one file for your reference.

One true story tells of a young woman who did not obtain the results of a Pap smear. She assumed that all was well since she had not heard from her doctor. In reality the physician did not receive the results from the laboratory. Since he had numerous patients, he didn't realize that this particular Pap interpretation was missing. Six months later the doctor was told that the Pap slide had been found. Unfortunately it showed that the young woman had cervical cancer, and she eventually died.

Physicians and patients need to take joint responsibility for any medical result. Be proactive and call your doctor if you don't hear back. That call may save your life!

TV

Can television program your kids? Studies have shown that there are about 20 to 25 acts of violence during an average hour of children's TV. Also, 60% of all television programs are violent. One study shows that the amount of time adolescents spent watching TV correlates strongly with aggressive acts directed against other people. As with the movie theaters, more parental controls are needed to help our children make the proper viewing choices.

Very Helpful Phrases

I have found the following phrases to be useful in everyday life. I do not know the origin of such wisdom but acknowledge the brilliance that these sentences convey.

The right word spoken at the right time sometimes achieves miracles.

A wish changes nothing. A decision changes everything.

The two best words in the English language: thank you.

The trail is the thing, not the end of the trail. Travel too fast and you miss all you are traveling for.

Giving is what makes our lives truly worthwhile.

If you don't have anything good to say about another person, don't say it.

Stress is when your gut says "no way" and your mouth says "sure, no problem."

Yesterday is history, tomorrow is a mystery and today is a gift.

I hope you find these phrases useful as well. Being polite, taking time to smell the roses, acting on positive ideas and giving to others sounds like good advice.

Chapter Six

Men's and Women's Health

Yes, we all know that men and women are different. My 20 years of practicing medicine has verified this fact. Some of these issues are so personal that you may not wish to tell your physician about them. Come out of the closet! Get personal with your physician since there is help available for these problems. We cannot cure the ailment if you don't tell us what ails you.

Benign Prostatic Hypertrophy

As the prostate grows larger with age, it starts to obstruct the bladder from emptying properly. One gets dribbling, slow-stream urination at night, and hesitancy. Thirty-five percent of all men will need surgery or medications.

Since the prostate is 80% muscle, alpha blockers will work quickly as they help relax the prostate muscle cells. (Examples enclude Hytrin, Cardura and Flomax.) Saw palmetto may be helpful to reduce the size of the prostate. Proscar reduces symptoms by decreasing prostate size, but takes about 12 months to work. It also reduces acute obstruction of the bladder by 57% and the need for surgery by 55%. Cardura can cause shortness of breath and should not be used if there is any evidence of heart failure. Flomax can often improve symptoms within 4 days and works more quickly than the other alpha blockers. Take this drug one-half hour after the same meal each day. This agent is also more costly than the other alpha blockers.

A combination of an alpha blocker such as Cardura (doxasosin) to relax the prostate and Proscar to shrink the prostate is a reasonable way to help this common problem. Interestingly, in clinical studies, this combination reduced the risk of progression by 67%. In other words, not only do the symptoms get better, but also benign prostatic hypertrophy may not even progress.

Erectile Dysfunction

This problem can occur due to smoking, stress, depression, medication, too much alcohol, poor circulation, prostate surgery, high LDL or bad cholesterol, neurologic disorders and decreased testosterone levels (often accompanied by poor libido, fatigue, decreased strength, depression and weaker bones).

Smoking is the number one cause of erectile dysfunction since it clogs up the circulation.

If you have early-morning erections or can have erections with other partners or by viewing erotic materials, then there is likely a psychosocial problem. Twenty percent of men have a psychological problem associated with erectile dysfunction, while 80% have an organic problem.

Most of the physical problems are associated with poor blood flow to the penis. Thirty million men between the ages of 40 and 70 suffer from impotence. Fifty-two percent of men note a change in their erections between ages 40 and 70.

If you notice that your desire for sex is reduced, you may be suffering from hypogonadism, or low testosterone. Depression needs to be ruled out first. Once this is done, a testosterone level should be obtained. If the level is below 400 nanograms per deciliter, further testing is needed.

Viagra represents an excellent treatment for erectile dysfunction. It works within 45 minutes and will require stimulation by your partner. This drug is effective 50 to 90% of the time, depending on the type of illness. Avoid Viagra if you are taking nitroglycerin or have active heart disease. Viagra is safe to take if you have heart disease, exercise regularly and are not having cardiac symptoms. Do not take Viagra with food as it impairs absorption. Other treatments include vacuum devices and rings, which are available over the counter. Injectable devices can also be used (Caverject). This device is injected with the click of a pen into the penis. The medicine helps to open up the arteries in the penis. Arginmax (includes arginine, ginkgo and ginseng) improved the ability to maintain erections in 88% of men in a small study. It is available over the counter. Androgel, a topical testosterone gel, and testosterone injections can be effective if the man has a low testosterone level. Counseling may be needed if a psychosocial problem is present. Penile implants are usually a final option for erectile dysfunction.

Estrogen

This hormone can help add 3 years on to your life when used without progesterone. The risk of breast cancer is negligible, especially in the first 5 years of usage. After that time, the risk of breast cancer increases by 35%, or 2 additional patients out of every 1,000. This drug may also help with depression, diabetes, osteoporosis and the prevention of both colon cancer and Alzheimer's. It definitely increases bone density. It is not helpful in the treatment of Alzheimer's.

Whether it helps in heart disease is debatable at this time. Do not begin estrogen if you have a history of coronary artery disease, as it may aggravate this problem. With its use the HDL cholesterol is increased, which is helpful, but the triglycerides (fats) are increased, which is a negative. Also estrogen increases CRP, a risk factor for heart disease.

Estrogen and progesterone have also been studied together. A study entitled the Women's Health Initiative (WHI) showed that lung clots were doubled after 5 years of treatment with an estrogen-progesterone combination. Additionally, there was a 41% increase in stroke, a 29% increase in heart attacks, a 26% increase in invasive breast cancer and a 22% increase in overall heart disease. Estrogen is useful for the treatment of menopausal mood swings, vaginal dryness, etc. If one is having menopausal symptoms, adding estrogen and progesterone can be very helpful in alleviating symptoms. The risk of breast cancer increases after 4 years, and the risk of heart attacks and strokes begins in the first 2 years of treatment.

One approach might be to use this combination during the first 2 years of menopause. After that time, the symptoms may have lessened and the hormones can be withdrawn. Other drugs can be used for osteoporosis prevention and treatment if necessary.

Estrogen is not ordinarily used alone as it can induce the production of uterine tumors. If you don't have a uterus, estrogen could be used for long periods of time since the above clinical trial did not study estrogen alone. Progesterone protects against cancer of the uterus, but causes other problems as previously stated. Discuss the benefit and risk of these hormones with your physician.

Hair Growth

Excessive hair growth is generally genetic. Ovarian problems, such as polycystic ovary syndrome and adrenal gland problems, can contribute to abnormal hair growth. Medications such as Dilantin may occasionally play a role.

Treatment may include spironolactone, the birth control pill, etc. Vaniqa is the first prescription drug for unwanted hair. It stops an enzyme that causes hair growth. It may take 8 weeks or longer for visible improvement and it helps 50% of women. Hair removal by electrolysis is also effective.

Hair Loss

A study using Propecia showed that 1 mg a day for 5 years preserved or increased hair growth in 65% of men. This drug is approved for the treatment of male-patterned baldness and may cause reversible erectile dysfunction in 2% of men. It works for frontal and top-of-the-head hair loss. Once the drug is stopped, hair loss will resume.

If a woman develops male-patterned hair loss (at the top of the head and front) especially after menopause, treatment may consist of Minoxidil spray twice daily. Minoxidil is also approved for use in men. Propecia is not approved for women.

Diffuse hair loss or shedding (telogen effluvium) commonly occurs in women and hardly ever results in baldness. Most women, however, find the hair loss alarming. Eighty-five percent of our hair is in a growing phase at any particular time. All it takes is a trigger to cause our hair to go into a resting phase for 3 to 6 months. These triggers, which can cause shedding, include hormonal changes, post pregnancy, fever, anesthesia, drugs, emotional stress, vegetarian diets, major surgery, infection, chronic illness, autoimmune diseases, early male-patterned baldness and nutritional deficiencies. Primary treatment consists of time and removal of any ongoing triggers. Finally, B complex vitamins (containing 3 to 5 mg of biotin B7), oral steroids, spironolactone and the birth control pill may be helpful.

Other causes of hair loss may include medications (Coumadin, cancer chemotherapy, progesterone, lithium, methotrexate, valproic acid, etc.), obsessive pulling of the hair, infections and autoimmune diseases (lupus and alopecia areata).

Hot Flashes

Menopause may cause these symptoms. Estrogen can help and is the gold standard. Additional treatments include the following: soy (40 to 60 grams of soy protein daily), vitamin E (400 to 800 units daily), progesterone, Effexor XR and Paxil (Effexor XR and Paxil are antidepressants approved for hot flashes). Infections, anxiety, thyroid disorders and rarely tumors also can cause hot flashes.

Black cohosh, an alternative medicine, seems to decrease hot flashes. Consider Remifemin, a form of black cohosh that has been used in clinical studies. Chastberry, evening primrose oil, dong quai and wild yam probably do not help.

Libido Disorders in Women

Causes to be considered include pain (from infection, tumors, endometriosis, lack of lubrication), psychological (poor partner interaction, depression, anxiety, abuse, religious issues), other diseases (diabetes, stroke, incontinence, drugs) and hormonal imbalance.

Testosterone is produced by the ovaries and adrenal glands. By measuring testosterone levels and DHEA-S (a precursor of testosterone made by the adrenals) your doctor can determine whether you have a deficiency. Testosterone deficiency in men and women can cause decreased libido and fatigue and possibly osteoporosis.

Treatment in a woman may include Estratest (a combination of estrogen and methyltestosterone for postmenopausal women), Androderm (a testosterone patch), DHEA (over the counter and often started at 50 mg per day, according to your testosterone and DHEA-S levels) and possibly Androgel (a topical testosterone gel). All of these treatments would be considered experimental and should be discussed with your physician.

Marriage

More than 50% of marriages do not succeed. There is no magic plan for success, but there are certain guidelines that may help.

1) As we age, each of us changes, therefore friendship should form the basis of a good marriage. While sex may indeed be important in a relationship, friendship provides the commitment necessary for a prosperous marriage.
2) Your spouse must be number one in your life. Both of you are team USA! Family and friends are the hospitable nations. If your actions convey that your mom, dad, sister, or brother come first, your partner will most certainly be hurt.
3) Communication is very important in all marriages. Talk honestly with each other and be a good listener. Communicate your needs, desires and dreams. Don't dwell on money matters and negative events. What do you want from your spouse? (Listen and find out.) This is a great place to start. Also, remember to talk about common interests and happy times.
4) Take vacations and spend more time together. Cultivate your friendship and become more intimate. Don't take marriage for granted. The flower won't grow without sunshine and water. If taking time with each other isn't a priority in your marriage, it most certainly will fail.
5) Follow through with your responsibilities. Remember that marriage is a partnership, a joint venture. If you both are healthy, divide the duties. Learning how to do each other's tasks can be illuminating and helpful. If one of you gets sick, for example, the other spouse then can be helpful instead of helpless.
7) Get ready to compromise. Don't get caught up in trivia. Win-win solutions are the best. A little give and take

can work wonders for your marriage. Don't try to fully control the other partner.

8) Be accountable for your actions. A fundamental human trait is to blame others when the proper results aren't achieved. Don't blame your spouse for your bad day at work. You created the experience, hence you need to take credit for it. Own up to it and get on with your life.

9) Take care of yourself. It is hard to have a partnership if you don't strive to keep yourself well. Exercise, eat right, take vitamins, obtain a physical exam, obtain psychotherapy, enjoy your vacations, etc.

10) I think you get the point. Marriage is a business and should be treated as one. It can be the best business in the whole world or your worst nightmare. Just like running a business, marriage requires compromising, fair task-sharing, good communicating, making friends, prioritizing, and keeping yourself in good health.

Parenting

One of the biggest domestic problems that this nation faces is the breakdown of the family unit. Marriage and parenting cannot adequately be covered in the home. Perhaps our schools could offer more courses in these important areas. Here are some general rules about parenting that may help to build a stronger family unit.

1) You are your kids' parents, not necessarily their friends. It's easy to be a friend, and it's hard to tell your kids what they do not want to hear. This concept also applies when your parents become old and are unable to care for themselves. At that time the parent-child role often reverses. For example, perhaps your parents don't want to go to an assisted living facility when it is clear that living at home is not safe anymore. This is not a time to tell your parents what they want to hear. It is a time to

move them in the direction of doing what's clearly best for them.

2) What you do is much more important than what you say. If you are drinking, smoking, using alcohol and marijuana, you won't be able to hide it, and your kids will pay more attention to your actions. You will no longer have any credibility with them. You are your child's best role model. Don't expect the latest sports hero to set the standard for your kid.

3) Pick your battles. Fighting over every small issue is grounds for a miserable household. You may wish to fight over drugs, driving safely, sexual issues and trust, rather than an ear piercing or a radio station.

4) Have a family meeting a few times a year and keep notes. Let your child talk, and be a good listener about what bothers him or her. Parents, write down some ground rules about household responsibilities for your children, and write down any other pressing issues. Talk to them candidly about drugs, sex, drinking, school, trust, smoking, etc. Please don't take it for granted that your kids understand these issues. If you don't communicate your viewpoints, they may assimilate the views of their peers. Laugh and joke a bit and attempt to form some conclusions. Refer back to these notes when your child says, "You never told me that." Have monthly meetings; you'll be surprised how effective these family conversations can be.

5) Don't let your child split you as parents. Both parents should fully agree on important issues so that a uniform approach is taken. Don't fall for "Daddy, look what Mom made me do." Talk to your spouse first before you agree with your child.

6) Be careful about abuse. Hitting your kids and making idle threats like "clean up your room or else" serves no purpose. Verbal abuse can be equally bad, for example, correct your children, but don't tell them that they are

worthless or stupid. Be positive about their good efforts and accomplishments. Try the following game; it really works! Tell your son or daughter to name all your personal strengths and then do the same for them. This is an all-around positive experience and esteem builder for your child.

7) Eat at least one meal together daily and communicate. Listen to their complaints, and don't be so quick to give immediate opinions. When they want to talk, drop everything and listen!

8) Try not to shield your child from life. Build trust by never lying. (You may wish to be selective in your words.) Take your kids to funerals, tell them when a family member is sick, encourage your child to work part-time. In other words, if your child wants a car, don't hand it to him or her on a silver platter. Give them a taste of life. Have them work toward a down payment on the car and perhaps you pay for the rest.

9) Parenting is also like a business, but it's a bit different from the business of marriage. If you micromanage and overcontrol your children's lives, you may end up with a rebellious kid who has an eating disorder. On the other hand, if you fail to communicate your views and correct mistakes, you may end up with a kid who abuses drugs and has unprotected sexual intercourse. If you consider the above rules and maintain the right parental balance, a child's inner beauty will shine. Equally important, these fine traits are more likely to propagate to the next generation. Good parenting can have an enormous effect on society for many generations after you're gone. That's what I call real leverage!

Premenstrual Syndrome

This syndrome occurs in 3 to 8% of all U.S. women. Fluctuating hormone levels probably account for the symptoms of this disease. Often symptoms begin 1 week before menstruation and may include irritability, mood swings, headache, breast swelling, edema and bloating.

Sarafem or Prozac at 20 mg a day continuously or just for two weeks prior to menses helps about 80% of women with this chemical disorder. It has FDA approval for continuous treatment. Zoloft also works and is approved at 50 to 100 mg for the 2 weeks prior to menstruation.

Additional therapies include aerobic exercise, calcium (1,200 mg per day of elemental calcium), vitamin E (400 units daily), diuretics for fluid retention (such as spironolactone at 100 mg daily beginning 2 weeks prior to menses), oral contraceptives (for headaches and breast tenderness) and Xanax for anxiety.

Sexually Transmitted Diseases (STD)

1) HPV, or the human papilloma virus, is the most common STD. Most people do not know that they have the virus. The virus may manifest as a fleshy wart on the genitalia. Removal does not eliminate the virus. Persistence of the virus can cause cervical cancer. Ninety percent of women will clear the virus in 2 years. Condoms help but do not prevent the disease. HPV is invisible and can be all over the genitals. Condoms only protect what is covered. The best prevention is abstinence. The Pap smear is the best screening test in women. Acetic acid can be applied to the male genitalia to expose warts. Often a white color will occur where the warts are located.

2) Chlamydia is a bacteria that can cause infertility, pelvic inflammatory disease and ectopic pregnancy in women. The disease can infect the testicle and cause infertility in men. The bacteria can travel up the female genital tract and scar the fallopian tubes. Seventy-five percent of women and 50% of men have no symptoms. Both

men and women can have burning on urination as well as a discharge from the penis or vagina. Chlamydia cultures to detect this disease can be done in the doctor's office. A special urine test is also effective in diagnosing chlamydia. Condoms, when used properly, are quite helpful in preventing this disease. Antibiotics such as azithromycin and doxycycline are effective in the treatment of this disease. Sexually active women especially between the ages of 18 to 25 should be screened since the complications of chlamydia can be devastating.

3) Herpes is a virus that causes recurrent blisters on the genitalia. Forty million people in the USA are infected. The first outbreak is painful and subsequent infections are usually mild. Both men and women frequently do not have any sores, yet they can still be infected with the virus and transmit it sexually. Treatment with Valtrex or Famvir or Zovirax (acyclovir) can shorten the course or prevent recurrent outbreaks. There is, however, no current cure. Condoms are helpful for prevention but since 50% of women shed the virus anywhere on the genitals, it can still be transmitted. This intermittent shedding of the virus occurs without symptoms. Genital herpes can be transmitted to the child during childbirth, so a cesarean section is needed in these individuals. Valtrex can help to decrease herpes transmission by 50%; however, the drug must be taken every day.

4) The three previously listed STDs are the most common ones seen in the USA. Other common sexually transmitted diseases include syphilis, HIV, gonorrhea, vaginal infections and hepatitis B. If you are diagnosed with an STD, your partner(s) should be informed and see his or her physician. Additionally, you should be tested for other STDs including HIV. Finally, condoms are helpful but far from perfect. Condoms will reduce HIV transmission by 85% and help prevent gonorrhea

in men. For the other STDs condoms are of unproven value, but probably helpful. Abstinence and a monogamous relationship are your best bets for safety at this time.

Urinary Incontinence

This problem affects more than 20% of adults. Stress incontinence is the most common type and results in the loss of urine with coughing or sneezing. Treatment includes the Kegel exercises (contracting the vaginal and rectal muscles for 1 to 2 seconds and then relaxing; do this 30 to 50 times a day), which works 75% of the time. Estrogen, collagen implants (a protein is injected around the urethra to give it support so you don't lose urine when you cough) and pads also can be useful.

Overactive bladder is also common and results in frequent small-volume urinations, particularly at night. The bladder just contracts too much. Bladder retraining is useful and involves gradually scheduling urinations farther apart. Utilize the Kegel exercises to help avoid frequent urinations. Medications such as Detrol LA and Ditropan XL can help decrease the frequent bladder contractions and incontinence. Detrol seems to have less dry mouth and central nervous system side effects.

Overflow incontinence usually results when the bladder is obstructed and is manifested by dribbling. In men it usually means that a large prostate is present. Sometimes diabetes and neurologic disorders may result in overflow incontinence, because the nerves to the bladder will not allow the bladder to contract.

With all incontinence make sure you see your doctor to rule out other causes including urinary infection, stool impaction, acute confusion, atrophic vaginitis, psychiatric problems, a dropped bladder, tumors, medications and neurologic problems.

Vacations

The Suny study showed that men who took at least annual vacations are 20% less likely to die over the following 9 years compared with men who didn't. Call your travel agent!

Chapter Seven

Mind Chemistry

Our nerve cells are like quarterbacks and receivers. The footballs are the hormones that allow communication between nerve cells. Anxiety, bipolar illness, depression, panic and posttraumatic stress disorder all have a chemical basis in the brain. Often a hormone is too low and needs replacement. This can even be demonstrated by a special functional scan of the brain called a PET scan. Improve your mind chemistry and you can improve your overall well-being. Once you take care of yourself you can begin to form successful relationships.

Anxiety

Symptoms include restlessness, irritability, insomnia, palpitations, breathing problems, stomach distress, frequent urination, etc.

Thyroid disease and other medical conditions must be ruled out. Treatment can include Paxil and Effexor XR, which are nonaddicting, exercise, psychotherapy, and benzodiazepines (Ativan, Xanax and Klonopin), which are potentially addicting).

Separate categories of anxiety include performance anxiety (fear of performing under observation; helped by Paxil), posttraumatic stress disorder (an anxiety state that often follows war, abuse, etc.; helped by Zoloft) and phobias (such as fear of heights).

Bipolar Disease

About 2 million people are affected and a genetic component exists. This disease usually manifests in the late teens and can be associated with suicide, substance abuse, impulsivity and poor judgment. Often these people become depressed, then have episodes of mania.

Symptoms of mania include inflated self-esteem, pressure of speech, "I can do anything" behavior, little or no sleep needed, hypersexuality, risk-taking behavior, etc. Sometimes symptoms of marked grandiosity can develop with concomitant delusions, for example, "I am a king with special powers."

Forty percent of bipolar patients have elements of depression and mania at the same time. This type of bipolar illness is often treated with mood-stabilizing medications such as Tegretol and Depakote, whereas the first type is usually treated with lithium. Antipsychotics such as Zyprexa can be helpful in both types of bipolar illness.

Sometimes when antidepressants are used alone, manic behavior can be precipitated. In other words, 10% of depressed patients are bipolar. The manic episodes become noticeable when an antidepressant is given without a mood stabilizer.

Depression

Common symptoms include feeling down consistently for at least 2 weeks, not experiencing pleasure, difficulty in concentration, agitation, guilt, low energy, suicidal ideation, etc.

This illness is chemical and affects more than 30 million people in the USA. It is not a sign of weakness, since

Abraham Lincoln, Winston Churchill, and John Lennon, to name a few, had depression.

Certain medications, recent physical illness, stress, alcohol, genetics, low testosterone, menopause, vitamin B12 deficiency, pancreatic cancer, lymphoma and thyroid disease may contribute to depression. Therefore, a complete physical exam is important. Once other causes of depression such as thyroid disease are ruled out, treatment may commence with psychotherapy and antidepressants.

Treatment with medication should take place for at least 1 year. Most antidepressants take 2 to 6 weeks to work. Ninety-five percent of patients with this ailment can be significantly helped! The B vitamins may play an important role in helping depression. B complex may raise levels of SAMe, a chemical that has antidepressant properties and antiarthritic properties. SAMe is quite expensive and B vitamins are cheap! Estrogen (without progesterone) may be helpful in treating depression as well. Also, it is known that eating more fish correlates with lower depression rates.

Adding short-term psychotherapy to medication can greatly enhance the results. Light therapy may also be helpful for depression and seasonal affective disorder (where you become down especially during the winter time when sunlight has decreased). Regular exercise for 16 weeks in people over 50 was just as successful as antidepressant medication. Finally, if you have unexplained physical symptoms, an antidepressant may help. (See Appendix D for more information regarding anxiety and depression.)

Happiness

I may not have the magic answer, but I can certainly tell you what won't work. Money will not buy you happiness. Billionaires are just as happy or unhappy as the poor. Alcohol, sex and drugs provide only a temporary fix. Having pity on yourself due to your awful past experiences will give you some solace, but ultimately you will need to forgive the past to obtain happiness. Building up your weak traits won't buy happiness either. Here are my suggestions.

1) Forgive the past so that you can get on with your life and start enjoying it.
2) Become passionate about something. Passion is the road to joy. My passion about writing this book brings me great joy. What is your passion? All I can say is that you will know it when you find it! Focus on your strengths, not your weaknesses. Toss around a few ideas that cater to your fortes.
3) Focus on building strong relationships with other people. Having good relationships can make life more fulfilling. Spiritual relationships also can lead to happiness.

Human Needs

In order to understand human behavior, we need to comprehend the 3 basic universal human needs. Although it may be oversimplifying, the following provides a framework.

We all have the need to control, survive and be appreciated. Almost all human behavior is dependent on these 3 needs.

Control issues often take a center position in marriage. The wife may tell the husband to go see the doctor to cure his cough. The husband refuses. The wife says she cares, and the husband says not to worry. Both are jockeying for control and the issue is the husband's health.

Survival issues are also universal and may involve saving face, your business or even your life.

Finally, everyone wants to be appreciated. This is a basic universal need. A comedian needs to be appreciated by her audience, an employee needs to be appreciated by his boss, a child needs to be appreciated by his parents and so on.

Keep these needs in mind when you are interacting with your family, friends and business associates.

Life's Commandments

No, I'm not trying to modify or replace the Ten Commandments. Whether or not you believe in the Ten Commandments is entirely up to you. In the ball game of life, relationships are crucial. These commandments apply to other people and to other nations as well. Let's examine these truths with real-life examples.

1) You can't care for others effectively unless you first care for yourself. You are number one; never demote yourself. If you refuse to exercise, take medicine, get psychotherapy and care for yourself, you won't be very helpful to other people who need you. If your father has Alzheimer's and you micromanage his life without regard to yourself, you will likely pay a price. Caretakers have a higher mortality if they don't make time for themselves. In addition, their other relationships will often suffer. If you keep your body and mind in the best shape possible, you can strive to have optimal relationships with your family, friends and business associates. Functional relationships bring true joy to our lives.

2) Be accountable for your own actions. A fundamental trait of human nature is to blame others for your own faults. My plant didn't grow because the seeds were no good. I didn't get a raise because my boss didn't understand my value to the company. I don't talk to my brother because he embarrassed me at the party. Certainly accidents, sickness, etc., may be out of our control; much of the time, however, we are accountable. Maybe you didn't water the plant properly or gave it too much sunlight. Perhaps you never showed your boss

how you personally increased revenues for the company. Your brother may have embarrassed you at the party because you were unknowingly rude to his wife. Start taking at least some ownership for your problems. Owning up to your own actions generates trust and respect. It is not a sign of weakness.

3) You control to some extent how other people treat you. Classical conditioning plays a prominent role in relationships. Here are some realistic examples. Why does he always tease me? Why does my husband beat me? Why does my boyfriend always meet me at lunch 20 minutes late? In part the reasons stem from your reinforcing the wrong behavior. In a way we are like Pavlov's dogs: Behavior that gets reinforced will be repeated. Maybe you get teased because the other person enjoys seeing you whine. Stop whining and change your behavior, and the teasing may stop. Ignoring the teasing and seeking help through the appropriate channels may lessen or eliminate this adverse behavior. The wife may be abused because she is inadvertently reinforcing the husband's dominant behavior. Certainly there is no excuse for the husband's abusive behavior. Going to a shelter, calling the police, seeking counseling or a divorce may quell this awful behavior. Finally, you may be reinforcing your boyfriend's late behavior by putting up with it. Perhaps you need to say, "Our time together is valuable, so let's be prompt for lunch." If this doesn't work, then leave the restaurant after 10 or 15 minutes. The undesired behavior will unlikely occur again.

4) Forgive the past so you can get on with the present. If you were raped in the past, you most certainly don't need to literally forgive the other person for such an evil deed. Begin by forgiving yourself. Forgiveness is done for yourself, not necessarily for the other person. Forgiving means letting go of these emotions in order for you to gain peace and freedom. In some way we

need to acknowledge the past but not be drowned by it. With time, the rape victim acknowledges the past, regains her humanity and starts living again. This may take time and psychotherapy, but it is critical for future relationships.

5) Attitude isn't crucial but behavior is. Certainly positive attitudes can give us a sense of comfort and peace. Our behavior, however, shapes the person that we are. Taking action is crucial for accomplishing our goals. How about if two people have the same goal to write a book? Both of them dream about the feeling of accomplishment, but only one of them writes what ends up to be a famous novel. Once again, behavior or action is what really matters. If you wish to lose weight, a good attitude is helpful but action is crucial. Eating healthier foods and exercising four times a week are action strategies that can lead to success.

Panic

This is another chemical problem that is characterized by "attacks" that come out of the blue. Symptoms may include choking, nausea, palpitations, sweating, dizziness, flushing, tingling, a feeling that you want to scream or run, mind-body dissociation, a feeling like you're going to die, etc.

Panic often occurs at night or away from the house. It may lead to agoraphobia or a fear of open spaces. This ailment differs from anxiety as it comes out of nowhere. Usually people become anxious as a result of anticipating another panic attack.

Panic disorder responds very well to treatment with antidepressants. This problem is often mistaken for a heart attack. Avoid caffeine, decongestants and other stimulants, since these drugs may aggravate or cause a panic attack.

Drug withdrawal, thyroid disease, heart and lung

disorders also can duplicate the symptoms of a panic attack. Your doctor may wish to consider these ailments before making the diagnosis of panic disorder.

Posttraumatic Stress Disorder

This problem arises as a result of a very stressful event. The 9/11 attack by terrorists on the World Trade Center caused posttraumatic stress disorder in millions of people. Combat stress in men and physical or sexual assault in women are additional key causes of this syndrome.

Symptoms include flashbacks, nightmares and hyperarousal. Depression, insomnia, panic, substance abuse and fatigue can be associated with posttraumatic stress. Serotonin reuptake inhibitors such as Paxil and Zoloft can be quite helpful to treat this problem. Psychotherapy may be very useful for this syndrome.

Chapter Eight

Money Tips

There are two rules of investing. First, preserve what you have. Don't lose it all by failing to purchase insurance policies and asset protection plans. Second, increase your net worth by investing in a legal yet safe fashion. Sleep better by reading the following money tips. Always review these ideas with your financial adviser.

Art

You'll never appreciate art so much till you talk with Mike Kuschmann at 1-800-229-4322 (Fine Arts Ltd).

Imagine buying art at wholesale, and then donating it to your favorite institution at retail. Let's say you are in the 35% tax bracket and you buy $5,000 of art at wholesale and donate it to a school at the retail price of $20,000. Your tax write-off is 35% of $20,000, or $7,000. Your initial investment was $5,000. That's a 40% return on your money. If you are in a higher tax bracket, your rate of return increases.

Everybody wins, including the institution and your wallet. Kuschmann has a national reputation and makes the whole process a cinch. Talk to him and your accountant. Kuschmann can also obtain art, antiques and jewelry at wholesale, so if you see an item that you wish to acquire, call him. He is a frequent speaker at national investment conferences and has his M.B.A., M.A. and B.A. from Stanford University. I personally utilize his services.

Estate Plan and Insurance

At least make sure that you have health, homeowner's, life and automobile insurance at a bare minimum. Certainly you should have a will. Don't leave your inheritance up to the state.

Reserve a plot of land (grave) for yourself. Save the sanity of your family by planning ahead even though it isn't easy. Remember to keep organized records. Make sure your family knows where you keep them.

If you have more than $500,000 in assets in addition to your residence, consider asset protection. You must plan before a lawsuit is filed. It is very easy to get sued and lose all the money that you have saved over the years. Now is the time to get your estate in order and protect your assets. Talk with Lee Phillips or Clark Gardner at 1-888-806-1997. You may also wish to use a local estate attorney and asset protection lawyer.

Living Will

It makes sense to have your attorney draft this document saying that if your condition is deemed irreversible by your doctor, you do not wish to have any extraordinary means used to prolong your life.

Get this made before you are ill, when you can plan with a clear mind. Most people do not want to be on a ventilator and have countless numbers of tubes for a condition such as metastatic cancer that is incurable. Plan ahead. Give the document to your doctor to place in your chart. Also, tell your closest family members what is written in your living will in case your physician forgets that it is in the chart.

When you are sick, you may be unable to communicate your wishes. If you don't want to be resuscitated (heart shocked and a tube put down your throat and connected to a ventilator), specify whether or not you want the following: artificial feeding (via a tube), artificial hydration (with an IV), antibiotics, hospitalization, blood drawing and other tests. Some people may not want their heart shocked but still desire hospitalization, antibiotics, etc. Others may want comfort measures only (pain control, hospice, etc.), and decline hydration, feedings, hospital care and the like.

In this document, make sure that you designate an individual to make decisions with regard to your health care should you be incapable of doing so. This is called power of attorney. This can save a doctor and a family many days of controversy with regards to the particulars of your medical care. Pick a responsible, caring family member or friend for this important task.

Money

Wealth is not as important as health, right? Talk to people who don't feel well, and you'll find out how meaningless money is and how important family, friends, health and religion become. Nevertheless, money provides security and options, just not happiness. No matter whether you are rich or poor, studies show that the level of happiness is about the same.

Don't speculate with your money. Einstein said that there is nothing better than compound interest. If you wish to hit home runs, have a funny money account and invest 5% of your money and have fun losing it just like in Las Vegas! In your serious account, stocks are by far your best bet over the long term. It makes no sense to place all of your funds in a money market at 55, while even low inflation at 4% gives you a meager return. The following suggestions may help.

1) Consider choosing Charles Schwab. They are rated the best on-line brokerage firm by *Money* magazine, and they are a firm with good vision and execution.

2) Eighty-five to 90% of mutual funds can't even beat the S+P 500, a standard index of 500 stocks. These funds' managers are pros who visit companies and crunch the financial numbers of each company. Do you think you can do better over the long term while managing your own career? Invest in an index fund such as the S+P 500. Make sure it has a low expense ratio and just park it there. The tax consequences will be small because there will be little turnover in stocks, and you will do better than 90% of investors. If you wish to invest in a mutual fund that is not based on an index, look at who is managing it. If Warren Buffet is managing my fund, I don't give a hoot if he has a down year. I know that he has a fantastic track record over the long term.

3) *The Spear Report* is an interesting newsletter that takes the best stock pickers according to Hulbert, the guru on financial newsletter performance. The highest rated stock is the one that most or all savvy stock investors pick (1-800-491-7119).

4) *How to Retire Rich* is an excellent quick read by James O'Shaughnessy. He is a scientist and divulges sound, safe strategies that have beaten the S+P 500 for nearly half a century. If you don't have a lot of time to spend, read this book and invest in his funds and be disciplined. Leave the money alone! It is so tempting to sell mutual funds when there is a significant drop; however, what the crowd does is not in your best interest. Know yourself before you invest. Can you sleep at night if your mutual fund drops 15%? If you are disciplined and controlled, the above advice will prove helpful. Alternatively, you can set your loss limit at 20 to 25%. Sell your investment when this limit is reached and don't

look back! In most cases the stock will continue to go lower. Love is for relationships, not for stocks.

5) Do you want zero downside and unlimited upside? Consider investing in MITTS (Market Index Target-Term Securities). MITTS were created by Merrill Lynch and can be purchased on-line or by your broker in virtually any market index such as the S+P 500 or the Nikkei index. When you buy these issues as they come out, you cannot lose your principal as long as you keep your investment for the term of the MITTS. The term may be up to 6 years depending on when you purchased it. If the index goes up, you can receive almost the full-percentage gain. These investments trade like stocks, and you can sell earlier than 6 years if you have a nice gain. If you have a big loss in 3 years, for example, you can always wait the entire 6 years and you will recover your principal. You will even make more if the index goes higher than your initial purchase. MITTS start at 10 dollars per share when they are first issued. If you buy 100 shares, you can't lose the $1,000 if you wait until maturity. If it goes up to $20 a share, you can receive 80 to 90% of the gain. Bullet-proof your portfolio with MITTS like I have. Give Lee Phillips a call at 1-800-806-1997. His capable financial staff will advise you how to proceed with this superb strategy.

There are also mutual funds that promise to protect your principal investment (not dividends). The family of funds called Pilgrim does this. There are higher internal fees, but you'll probably sleep better at night.

6) Check out these suggestions with your financial adviser. Most important, pick a strategy that makes you comfortable from the psychologic standpoint. This is absolutely crucial. Buy-and-hold really works, but how long can you hold if a bear market strikes for years? The market has a habit of finding out your own personal

weaknesses. I have no financial relationship with the above authors.

Prescription Drug Costs

Save money by shopping on line, for example, drugstore.com, or purchase medicines out of the country such as from Canada. You may save up to 75%. For instance, www.canadameds.com offers prescription medicines at significant discounts. Talk to your lawyer regarding the current laws concerning this before purchasing.

Also, if you are a veteran, try your local VA and save a bundle. In addition, most pharmaceutical companies have patient-assistance programs and dispense free medication if you qualify.

Finally, split higher-dose pills with a pill splitter and once again save money. For example, if you take a 20 mg pill, often the 40 mg won't cost twice as much, so it's cheaper to split them. Ask your pharmacist if it is safe to do this since some drugs have special delivery systems that could be hampered by cutting the pill in half. Obtain an inexpensive pill splitter at your local drugstore.

VEBA

One should always max out his or her retirement plan to get tax-deferred money at a later date. Remember, Einstein said that compound interest is the best invention. If you have done a retirement plan or can't do one, consider a VEBA (Voluntary Employees' Beneficiary Association). What does this plan allow?

1) Almost unlimited annual contributions can be made.
2) All contributions are fully tax deductible and compounding occurs in a tax-free environment.
3) Contributions to the plan buy benefits. If the benefit

purchased is a life insurance vehicle, you can control where cash values are invested. Therefore you build up cash rapidly in a tax-free environment. Additionally you have excellent life insurance. Cash values can be used to pay for additional benefits including medical, nursing home, education, disability, etc.

4) The plan provides for nearly complete asset protection.

5) The life insurance can go to your beneficiary free of income and estate tax.

If you are in a 25% tax bracket or higher, give Lee Phillips, an attorney before the U.S. Supreme Court, a call at 1-800-806-1997. Talk to your accountant and have him or her talk to Mr. Phillips to help you set up this plan and make sure it is appropriate for you. I find him reputable and trustworthy.

Chapter Nine

Personal Habits

Here are a few items that can enrich the quality of your life.

Botox Injections

It's ironic that botulinin toxin can be deadly in the disease called botulism, yet that very same toxin can work miracles if utilized by a skilled physician. Botox can can cause relaxation of muscles and alleviate migraine headaches, overactive bladder, tremors associated with Parkinson's disease, contracted muscles due to strokes and laryngitis due to spasm of the vocal cords (spasmodic dysphonia). Botox injections usually last 3 to 6 months. This medicine also can be used to decrease wrinkles, but it is expensive. The most common side effect is temporary weakening of surrounding muscles as the toxin spreads from the original site of injection. Avage, Retin-A and Renova are all topical retinoids that also can be used to lessen wrinkles but need to be applied daily. Remember to focus on prevention by avoiding ultraviolet light.

Breakfast

For some reason people who do not eat breakfast have 1.5 times the mortality rate of individuals who eat breakfast regularly. Fruits, grains and fiber probably contribute to a healthier lifestyle.

Dogs

Owning a dog just might save your life. There is also evidence that other pets can be helpful too. One study shows that after a heart attack, dog owners have an increased survival as compared to people who do not have a pet.

Perhaps the act of walking the dog is beneficial or maybe loneliness is reduced. Stroking your pet likely produces good hormones in the body. This is presently being studied. "Man's best friend" may indeed be a reality!

Flossing

Help to prevent gingivitis and periodontal disease with flossing on a regular basis. A Center of Disease Control study indicated that people with gum disease have a 23 to 46% higher mortality rate than the average population.

Apparently such individuals have a higher incidence of heart disease, stroke and infections. Perhaps the plaque that builds up on the teeth also accumulates in our arteries. Therefore, brush your teeth and floss on a regular basis.

I find that an electric flosser is fast and easy. This gadget almost makes flossing fun, rather than a chore.

LASIK

This stands for laser-assisted in-situ keratomileusis. This procedure is the most commonly performed refractive surgery and helps to correct mild, moderate or severe nearsightedness with or without astigmatism. Farsightedness may be treated as well.

The eye doctor uses a microkeratome to create a flap of cornea. (The device is used like a carpenter's plane.) Once the flap is made, the surgeon uses an excimer laser to thin the corneal flap precisely. It is then sutured back in place. The recovery is quick and there is very little discomfort. Both eyes can be done in the same day.

More than 90% of patients are satisfied with this procedure, and corneal-flap complications are infrequent. This procedure corrects distance vision, but does not correct reading vision. Avoid this procedure if you have diabetes, cataracts, corneal disease, poor immunity, uncontrolled vascular disease, keloids or autoimmune disease. Also avoid LASIK during pregnancy or while nursing.

Nurse Practitioners and Physician Assistants

Both of these professionals assist physicians in the care of their patients. They may see patients independently of the physician. Generally they review patient cases with the on-site physician. Often their care is exceptional because they take extra time to listen to their patients. Additionally, they can prescribe medicines.

Physician Issues

Choosing isn't an easy matter but here are a few pointers. It is very important that your doctor be board certified. This doesn't guarantee that your doctor is an excellent physician, but it helps. This is a rigorous exam that 40 to 50% of doctors fail. Around 1985 new physicians were required to update their board certification every 10 years.

Does your doctor do continuing medical education (CME)? Each state has its own requirements. (You can find this out from the AMA.) Doing CME ensures that your doctor is at least attempting to keep up-to-date.

Will your personal physician allow you to interview him or her for 10 minutes at no charge? If the physician does not allow a short interview, then be suspicious that the doctor is too busy or has a big ego. During the interview ask about board certification, CME issues, waiting time to get an appointment, average waiting time in the reception room, same-day callbacks, cross coverage with other doctors, hospital affiliations, nursing home affiliations, etc. Is the doctor friendly and empathetic or cold and dictatorial? Does the doctor have multiple offices and hospital affiliations? Does the doctor do research and lecture nationally? If so, will there be enough time left for you?

The physician's bedside manner is just as important as the knowledge base. Doctors make diagnoses primarily by what you say as opposed to the examination and labs. If you are uneasy with your physician, you are less likely to reveal information about sensitive issues such as stress, depression, drugs, erectile dysfunction, etc.

By the way, it doesn't matter if you are being seen by an MD or a DO (doctor of osteopathy). In my opinion, these are equivalent degrees.

When you see your doctor always bring a list of medications, remind him or her of any allergies and bring a list of your problems. Please be reasonable. If you bring a list of 5 complaints, don't expect the physician to do a thorough job in 15 minutes. That's only 3 minutes per complaint! Schedule a longer visit if you have a lot of questions. Remember to do periodic exams even if you feel well. Blood pressure, cholesterol, cancer and heart disease all can be silent problems.

Call your doctor after hours if you feel you have an emergency. Make sure that you make appointments, address billing issues and refill prescriptions during regular office hours.

Sometimes patience wears thin when you're ill, but be courteous to the staff. If there is a problem, most offices have an office manager who usually can help you with an issue. Also, never stay with an inadequate physician because you're scared that you might hurt his or her feelings. Your health comes first.

Finally, feel free to get a second opinion from a specialist about a puzzling problem. Your doctor is there to help assist you in your care. The physician's ego is secondary.

Self-Exam

Consider doing a testicle self-exam. This is the most common cancer between the ages of 18 and 45. Feel for a firm small nodule on the testicle monthly.

The breast self-exam should be done monthly in the shower while the breasts are soapy, since nodules can be felt more easily.

Examine your skin monthly for moles, especially ones that are multicolored, irregular or growing. A new change in a mole is also an early warning sign. Use a mirror to check the nape of the neck, bottom of the feet, etc.

Finally, don't use cotton swabs in your ears. They just push wax farther into the ear canal.

Sex

A recent study from Great Britain shows that men who have sex more than the average of once per week have lower mortality from all causes! Having sex 1 to 2 times a week will increase immunoglobulin A, an antibody that fights respiratory infections. More sex did not enhance the immune system further.

Certainly, HIV, herpes, HPV, gonorrhea, syphilis, hepatitis B, chlamydia and unwanted pregnancy are the downside. Use condoms and maintain a mutually monogamous relationship.

Sleep

A study from Alameda County in California shows that men who sleep 7 to 8 hours nightly and women who sleep 6 to 7 hours nightly have lower mortality rates. Sleep decreases stress, enhances attention span and boosts the immune system.

Most sleeping pills are potentially addicting. Ambien and Sonata work quickly for sleep and have a very low incidence of addiction. Possible natural sleep aids include valerian (150 to 300 mg of a standardized extract containing 0.8% valeric acid; take 30 minutes before bedtime) and melatonin (0.5 to 6 mg at bedtime). Avoid these supplements if you have lymphoma, leukemia, severe allergies, pregnancy or depression. Trazadone, a nonaddicting antidepressant, can also be helpful (dizziness, prolonged drowsiness and persistent erection may occur). Benadryl and alcohol are poor sleeping agents. By the way, Benadryl is just as dangerous as alcohol when one drives a motor vehicle. Benadryl (diphenhydramine) is available over the counter.

It is very important to find the cause of insomnia so specific treatment can be instituted. The most common causes include psychiatric (depression and anxiety), physiologic (thyroid disease, medications, caffeine, alcohol, menopause, urinary problems, heart failure, etc.) and psychophysiologic. Interestingly, many people use the bedroom for a host of activities besides sleep. Such individuals become conditioned not to sleep! This is called a psychophysiologic sleep disorder. If you are using the bedroom to work, watch TV, and eat, then you may just end up watching the clock all night. Utilize the bedroom for sleep and sex only. If you cannot sleep after 20 to 30 minutes, then get out of the bedroom and read in another room until you are sleepy again. This way, the bedroom becomes associated with sleep only. Avoid caffeine anytime during the day and exercise earlier in the day. Decongestants and diet pills are medications that commonly keep people awake at night. (See Appendix E for a review of the diagnosis and treatment of insomnia.)

Tooth Whitening

Whitening toothpastes are well tolerated and remove surface stains but do not make the teeth brighter. Bleaching products, such as Colgate Simply, actually do brighten the teeth. This particular product comes in gel form and needs to be applied twice daily for about 2 to 4 weeks. Tooth sensitivity is reported but usually goes away after treatment. Use as directed on the product since too much bleaching may cause tooth and gum damage. Dentists can apply higher concentrations of the bleaching agent and it will work faster. The procedure usually costs between $400 and $1,000. Bleaching removes only superficial brown or yellow stains. It does not remove stains that are deeper and gray colored.

Chapter Ten

Vaccinations

The right vaccine at the proper time can prevent a disease and save your life. The marked benefits of these medications almost always outweigh the small risks.

Chicken Pox Vaccine

This vaccine (varivax) is a live vaccine and should be given to healthy children at 12 months of age.

Young adults who have not had the disease should receive 2 shots at 1 to 2 months apart. This disease is more serious in adults due to respiratory and rarely brain complications.

Avoid the vaccine during pregnancy or if you are allergic to neomycin or gelatin. Avoid any immune globulin shots 2 months before or 5 months after this vaccine.

This vaccine can prevent chicken pox 90% of the time if a person has been recently exposed. Even if you do get the disease, it is almost always mild if the vaccination has been administered within 3 days of exposure. Varivax may still be effective if given within 5 days of exposure.

Flu Shot

If you are not allergic to eggs, are 50 or older, or if you're younger and have a chronic disease such as diabetes, heart disease or a respiratory disorder, get a flu shot.

You also may take it if you just don't want to lose time from work. Thirty thousand people die from the flu yearly in the USA (usually the elderly). Often it begins with fever and body aches. The disease can progress to pneumonia and even death.

In addition, if you live with an individual in poor health, you may wish to obtain the flu vaccine. This helps to protect that frail individual from developing influenza.

Side effects can include local reactions such as redness at the site of injection and rarely flulike symptoms for a couple of days. Avoid this vaccine if you have a high fever or if you are allergic to eggs or preservatives in the shot. You cannot get the flu from this vaccine as it contains dead virus.

Tamiflu, an oral agent, can reduce the duration of flu symptoms by more than 3 days, if it is started in the first 12 hours. It can still reduce the duration of this disease if it is given within the first 48 hours of onset. Take Tamiflu, 75 mg twice daily for 5 days with food. Flu symptoms are nonspecific and may include body aches, fever, diarrhea and cough. Most colds are not associated with fever and body aches. Sore throat, hoarseness, and sneezing are more frequent with the common cold. The American Academy of Family Practice now recommends flu shots if you are 50 or older. A flu test is available that detects about 75% of flu cases.

Pneumovax

Obtain this important vaccine under the same circumstances as a flu shot. This medicine protects against half of all pneumonias. It is given every 5 to 6 years beginning at age 2 if you have a poor immune system or a chronic disease such as heart failure, diabetes, asthma or emphysema. At age 65 or older, 1 pneumonia vaccination is sufficient for life. Beginning Pneumovax at age 50 and giving it again at age 65 even if there is no evidence of chronic disease is often recommended. Side effects are similar to those of the flu shot. Both the flu shot and Pneumovax are dead vaccines. Oral typhoid, chicken pox vaccine and oral polio are live vaccines and should be avoided in those who are pregnancy and people with poor immunity.

Tetanus Shot

Obtain this vaccination every 10 years to protect yourself against this fatal bacteria (rare). If you are cut by a dirty object, obtain a tetanus shot promptly unless the last vaccination was within 5 years. A primary series of tetanus shots is suggested if one was never administered in the past.

Travel

If you are traveling out of the country, let your physician know so that he or she can help make your trip safe.

Hepatitis A infects 1 in 50 unimmunized travelers. Hepatitis A vaccine is needed for most destinations except Canada, Western Europe, Australia, New Zealand and Japan. This virus is transmitted by food handlers who don't wash their hands (fecal/oral spread). Shellfish are another source. Begin the hepatitis A vaccine at least 2 to 4 weeks before departure. A booster dose 6 to 12 months later can give at least 20 years of immunity.

Hepatitis B is less common. One in one thousand unimmunized travelers become infected. Take the hepatitis B vaccine if you are at high risk or if you are going to endemic areas such as Africa, Asia, Middle East, Southern Europe and some tropical areas. It's usually given in 2 to 3 doses over 6 months. Hepatitis B is usually spread by dirty needles, sexual intercourse and rarely by blood transfusions and bites.

Typhoid fever infects one in three thousand unimmunized travelers to developing countries. Obtain the single-dose injectable dead vaccine (Typhim Vi), which is good for 2 years, or the four-dose live oral vaccine (Vivotif Berna), which is good for 5 years. Obtain these vaccinations 2 to 4 weeks before departure.

Yellow fever vaccinations are required to enter some countries in sub-Saharan Africa and tropical South America. This vaccine is available only at clinics designated by the state health department. The vaccination is good for 10 years.

Malaria prophylaxis is needed in many tropical areas. Chloroquine is no longer effective in most areas. Mefloquine (Lariam) resistance is also showing up in Southeast Asia. For most travelers, use Lariam, doxycycline, or Malarone (atovaquone and proguanil). Stop taking Lariam if psychiatric symptoms occur, such as depression, hallucinations or suicidal thoughts. Avoid Lariam if there is a history of psychiatric illness. Use doxycycline or Malarone instead.

Travelers' diarrhea doesn't require an antibiotic for prevention, just prompt treatment of the diarrhea. Use loperamide (Imodium) for mild cases. Save antibiotics for severe diarrhea with fever or bloody stool. Take ciprofloxacin (Cipro) 500 mg twice daily for 3 days to treat this disease.

General items to bring on your trip include Cipro (antibiotic for traveler's diarrhea—try 500 mg twice a day for 3 to 5 days if diarrhea occurs; 250 mg twice daily for 3 days will cover most urine infections, too), Imodium and Pepto-Bismol (for diarrhea), Afrin nasal spray and Sudafed (both are decongestants for the plane or if you get a cold), antifungal creams such as Lotrimin (especially if in humid environments), Z-Pack (antibiotic for respiratory infections), insect repellent, Bonine, Dramamine or ginger (for sea sickness), Diamox (for altitude sickness), etc. Let your physician know at least 1 month ahead of time before leaving the USA so vaccines and advice can be given.

Chapter Eleven

Vitamins and Herbs

Vitamins and herbs can be useful adjuncts to your overall health. Look at these agents as drugs and always consult your physician and pharmacist for side effects. Exercise, diet, stress reduction, preventive health care and physician visits take precedence over these agents. Pharmaceutical agents, which are FDA approved, are more thoroughly tested than vitamins or herbs. We need better standardization of these agents so that we are consuming what the label states.

Creatine

This supplement generates ATP or energy for the body and may result in less fat and more muscle. Perhaps supplementation will be helpful for bodybuilders or if you are training for a race. The recommended dosage is 5,000 mg (1 tablespoon of powder in water or juice) daily. I am not in favor of most bodybuilding supplements because the cost is usually not worth the benefit. Additionally, side effects can be an issue, which also applies to Creatine.

Derma Q-Gel Cream

This cream is marvelous for wrinkles. It has a unique delivery system that provides coenzyme, green tea and 20 other active ingredients to help your skin look youthful. It may help reduce the incidence of skin cancer as well. Purchase this outstanding product with a money-back guarantee by calling 1-866-775-7628.

A keloid is a buildup of thick scar tissue due to the overproduction of collagen during wound healing. A keloid may be reduced by having your physician inject steroids into it. Aldara cream has been shown to help prevent the recurrence of keloids once they are excised.

Echinacea

This herb seems to be particularly effective against colds and flu. It probably stimulates the immune system and can help reduce the severity of upper respiratory infections. In people with poor immune systems, consider taking it chronically. Rare allergic reactions have been reported. Clinical trials on this herb's efficacy have been mixed.

Flaxseed Oil

Flaxseeds along with walnuts, peanuts and macadamia nuts contain alpha linolenic acid, an omega-3 fatty acid, which may help to decrease triglycerides, fight cancer and reduce arthritic symptoms. Fish also contain omega-3 fatty acids.

Additionally, flaxseed oil contains lignans, a type of fiber that may have an anticancer effect. With each meal, 1,000 mg can be taken in capsule form.

Ginger

A small study demonstrated that ginger at 1 gram daily helped to reduce nausea in pregnant women. No adverse effects on pregnancy outcome were seen. This herb may also be useful for seasickness.

Ginkgo Biloba

This herb may help with memory in Alzheimer's. There is controversy about whether it works in normal people with mild memory impairment. A small study in people between 30 and 59 demonstrated better memory recall when given a single 120-mg standardized extract (look for 24% flavon glycosides and 6% terpene lactones). On the other hand, another study conducted in people over age 60 demonstrated no effect on cognition when given 40 mg of this herb 3 times a day. The above two studies were conducted in patients with normal to mildly impaired memory. Ginkgo may also improve memory in Alzheimer's disease.

Ginkgo can thin the blood; hence do not take with Coumadin, and discontinue 2 to 3 weeks before surgery. Rarely this herb may cause seizures, and epileptic patients may wish to avoid this agent.

Glucosamine

These supplements may decrease the progression of wear-and-tear arthritis, or osteoarthritis. This type of joint disease is more common in women and tends to involve the hips, knees, feet, tips of fingers and bases of thumbs. Loss of cartilage results in painful movement. Tylenol and moderate exercise are the main treatments.

Glucosamine may take 1 to 3 months to work at 1,500 mg per day in divided doses. This supplement may stimulate cartilage growth as opposed to anti-inflammatories. It also likely works as well as anti-inflammatories but without the stomach and kidney side effects. It may raise blood sugar; hence type 2 diabetics should have their blood sugar monitored.

Other therapies for this disease may include vitamins C and E, chondroitin (900 to 1,200 mg a day may help with minimal side effects), MSM (a cheap over-the-counter supplement at 1,000 mg twice a day), Synvisc (a series of 3 knee injections of a honeylike joint-fluid lubricant that may help with pain for up to 1.5 years) and SAMe (an expensive supplement that may help with joint pain and depression; taking 600 to 1,200 mg in divided doses may be helpful).

Grapeseed Extract

This is a powerful, well-tolerated antioxidant. It has perhaps 50 times the antioxidant potential of vitamin E.

This vitamin thins the blood, which may help to prevent heart attacks. It also strengthens the blood vessels at the same time, thus helping with leg edema. Grapeseed extract may help with allergies and arthritis. A reasonable dose would be 90 to 180 mg daily.

Green Tea

Here is an example of a first-rate herb that can reduce the risk of a heart attack by 44% and has a marked anticancer effect.

In one study, moderate to heavy consumers of green tea showed markedly reduced mortality rate due to heart attacks. Heavy consumption was defined as drinking more than 14 cups per week and moderate consumption equated to fewer than 14 cups per week.

I have found a type of green tea capsules where each capsule is equivalent to 5 cups of green tea (see www.advancedvitamins.com). Other capsules are available over the counter, but not all green tea capsules are alike. Some capsules contain only 1 cup of green tea, while other preparations contain more.

Studies in Japan demonstrate low mortality rates from cancer, especially in people who consumed 10 or more cups of green tea per day. Green tea contains powerful antioxidants called polyphenols. The preparation of green tea that I prefer (and take myself) is standardized and contains 250 mg of polyphenols, equivalent to about 4 to 5 cups of green tea in each capsule. EGCG, a specific polyphenol, inhibits growth of blood vessels into a tumor and may even hinder metastases (spread of a tumor to distant sites in the body).

In addition to addressing the number one and number two causes of death in the USA (heart attacks and cancer, respectively), green tea may also help you to lose weight. It seems to possess thermogenic properties and promotes the breakdown of fats by a mechanism unrelated to its caffeine content. (For more information on green tea, see Appendix F.)

Hawthorn

This herb confers an array of benefits for the aging heart. Heart-failure patients seem to benefit as it helps to contract the heart better. It also reduces clotting, mildly lowers blood pressure and dilates the coronary arteries.

A European study showed reduction in heart-failure symptoms such as leg edema, shortness of breath and fatigue. A standardized extract is recommended. Many people take it as a preventative.

Kava Kava

This is a common herb in the Caribbean that is used for anxiety and depression. Like Chinese herbs, this herb can cause liver failure and should be considered only after other standard approaches have been exhausted.

Kava kava seems to have a calming effect without affecting mental acuity. A daily dose equivalent to 180 mg of kavalactones should be adequate. The entire 180-mg dose of kavalactones taken at bedtime can help with sleep. Seven small double-blinded controlled trials showed that 60 to 240 mg of kavalactones 2 to 3 times a day helped with anxiety. Kava kava was used for periods ranging from 1 to 24 weeks. Few side effects were reported. Sporadic cases of liver failure have been seen, and this herb should be used with caution. High doses can have alcohol-like effects.

Panax Ginseng

This herb (Chinese or Korean ginseng) probably helps to improve the immune response, memory and blood sugar and decrease stress and fatigue. The active ingredients are called ginsenosides. Obtain only a standardized extract of 4 to 7% ginsenosides, and only use panax ginseng. Do not take if you have hypertension. This herb may cause headaches and possibly vaginal bleeding. It probably does not improve athletic performance. It seems to reduce bacterial counts in acute bronchitis.

Q-Gel

This is the outstanding vitamin supplement of the twenty-first century. It is actually a brand version of coenzyme Q-10. Q-Gel is undoubtedly the best preparation since it maintains much higher blood levels than conventional coenzyme preparations. This natural vitamin, which is in all our cells, has applications for the heart, brain, cancer, longevity and gum disease. (See Appendix G for more information.)

Saw Palmetto

Benign prostatic hypertrophy is quite common and affects 50% of men by age 60. Symptoms include slow stream, hesitancy, urinating at night and sometimes irritation upon urination.

Saw palmetto probably blocks the conversion of testosterone to dihydrotestosterone, which likely causes the enlargement of the prostate. It works similar to Proscar. (See Chapter 6.)

Try taking 320 mg of saw palmetto at bedtime for 2 months to see whether it works. Side effects are rare and include nausea.

Soy

This supplement contains isoflavones (phytoestrogens) such as genestein and daidzein, which may help thwart the growth of prostate and breast cancer cells. Additionally, the protein in soy (isolated soy protein) lowers cholesterol and triglycerides by 10%.

Soy also may help to relieve the symptoms of menopause such as hot flashes, vaginal dryness and irritability, since it is a phytoestrogen. Good sources include tofu, soy milk and soybeans.

At least 40 to 50 grams a day of soy protein would be optimal to lower cholesterol by 10%. We're not sure whether it is the protein or isoflavones contained in soy that is responsible for lowering cholesterol.

Its effect on breast cancer remains controversial. Soy protein has a modest effect upon menopausal symptoms.

St. John's Wort

This herb is prescribed ten to one over Prozac in Europe for depression. It helps patients with depression 70% of the time. Side effects are few and include nausea and rarely a skin rash when exposed to the sun. Taking 900 to 1,200 mg per day in divided doses of a standardized 0.3% extract can be helpful in treating this disease.

Do not combine with prescription antidepressants. This herb may cause cataracts and does interact with digoxin, a heart drug. Discontinue prior to surgery. Finally, this herb may reduce the effectiveness of the birth control pill and interacts with some HIV drugs.

St. John's wort probably does not work in moderate to severe depression. It is best to use this herb only in mild cases of depression.

Vitamin A and Beta Carotene

This vitamin is found in green, orange and yellow fruits and vegetables. It may help to diminish certain cancers and heart attacks. Avoid this vitamin if you are alcoholic due to effects on the liver and if you are a smoker (smoking plus vitamin A may increase lung cancers beyond smoking alone).

This vitamin may also block vitamin D's ability to help absorb calcium. Postmenopausal women not on hormone replacement should take 10,000 units or less of vitamin A.

Vitamin B Complex

This is an excellent vitamin, as it helps to prevent neural tube defects in the newborn. Additionally, it may help to prevent stroke and heart attacks by reducing homocysteine, a chemical in our blood that causes clogging of our vessels with cholesterol plaque. There is evidence that B vitamins can prevent coronary arteries from clogging up after angioplasty.

Three cups or more of coffee daily can raise homocysteine levels, whereas protein and vitamins (especially B6, B12 and folic acid) will lower this deadly chemical. Additionally, the B vitamins help to relieve stress and probably improve cognitive capacity.

Finally, folic acid, which is a B vitamin, helped to reduce colon cancer by 75% in women. Mega Multiple 85 is an excellent multiple vitamin because it has high dosages of vitamin B complex and it's cheap and easy to swallow. (See Appendix H.)

The Journal of the American Medical Association now recommends a multiple vitamin daily.

Vitamin C

This wonderful vitamin helps with tissue repair, may reduce heart attacks, decreases duration of colds by 33% (recommend 1,000 to 5,000 mg per day for colds), may increase HDL, or good cholesterol, and finally it might help to reduce cancers of the mouth, larynx, stomach and pancreas.

Vitamin C cream can also help to reduce wrinkles.

Linus Pauling took 18,000 mg daily but he had to increase it gradually. Consider taking 500 to 1,000 mg daily. Do greater doses cause atherosclerosis? One study demonstrates this possibility but much more proof is needed. Another study showed that an extra serving of fruit a day (more vitamin C) reduced overall mortality by 20%!

Vitamin E

This vitamin possibly can boost the immune system, delay institutionalization in Alzheimer's patients, relieve leg cramps, possibly decrease menopausal symptoms and fibrocystic breasts and decrease the incidence of aggressive prostate tumors.

Take the natural d-alpha vitamin E, not the cheaper dl-synthetic. Two studies published in early 2000 showed that 300 to 400 units per day did not decrease or increase heart disease and stroke. Also one study published in 2002 showed no effect of vitamin E at 200 units a day upon the frequency of upper respiratory infections. In dialysis patients, vitamin E at 800 units per day reduced the risk of stroke and heart attacks. While this vitamin may be helpful for the prevention and treatment of Alzheimer's and prostate cancer, it does not seem helpful for the prevention heart disease or respiratory infections.

Chapter 12

Wrapping Up

Please know that the above information is based on years of experience and reflects my opinions. Statements may not always represent the opinion of the Food and Drug Administration.

Always check with your doctor first when it comes to diagnosing or treating disease. I have tried to base most of the data on the latest scientific articles. Failure to follow the preventive protocols outlined in this book can result in dire circumstances and can have a negative impact on your health. Examples include failing to have a colonoscopy, Pap smear, flu shot, regular physical exam, etc., as indicated in this book.

Over the last 20 years of practicing medicine, I find that the biggest problems in this field include compliance, malpractice and health care access.

Noncompliance kills so many good people. All of us have different beliefs. Commonly patients will stop their medication without telling their health care provider. Often I find that a critical medication was stopped because the patient had an unrelated symptom. Sometimes patients don't believe their doctor. "Doc, I know when my sugar is high; I don't need to test it." If you don't agree with your doctor, have a discussion with him or her about both of your beliefs. Otherwise get a second opinion, but don't ignore your doctor's advice without further exploration.

Many patients are not only noncompliant about taking their medications but also resistant about modifying their own lifestyles. "I don't want a colonoscopy." "I just like good food." "The cigarette is my best friend." "I don't have time to exercise because I have three kids and a stressful job." "I forget to take my medicine at night."

I urge you to discuss these issues with your doctor. Change does indeed take time. Keep an open mind and never give up on yourself. For example, if you have a receptive doctor, you may decide not to do a colonoscopy this year but perhaps you will be ready the following year. The doctor needs to be receptive, but remember that he or she cannot control your actions. Your physician should assist you in caring for yourself, rather than dictating and making you feel badly. Discuss your feelings. Why are you afraid of this test? Why don't you like this medication? What are the barriers that keep you from exercising?

As to the problem of malpractice, doctors are human beings. Sometimes we make mistakes, but most of us care about our patients. A few health care providers have no conscience and don't keep up with the medical literature. Some of these individuals deserve to be sued. Most cases, however, should never be considered. Nationwide, more and more physicians are leaving the field due to rising malpractice premiums and frivolous lawsuits.

I suggest that additional required education is needed for physicians. Courses in empathy and the latest medical breakthroughs would make us all better health care providers. At the present time, continuing medical education is required by many states.

Some plaintiff attorneys are eager to take on a client's case because they smell the large cash rewards. I suggest that plaintiff lawyers should receive only 5 to 10 percent of the malpractice awards. This would get rid of the nuisance lawsuits, and only the cases of questionable malpractice suits would hit the courtroom. Many attorneys would protest such fixed lower percentages, but physicians' fees are already fixed and even being reduced by the government. Alternatively, patients could elect to pay their attorneys an hourly fee to prosecute a physician.

The most important issue in medicine, however, is that everyone should have health care access. Prescription coverage, physician care and hospital benefits for everyone can happen only when a task force is formed that includes physicians, pharmaceutical representatives, hospital administrators, governmental officials and insurance representatives. All of these groups will need to contribute their ideas to develop a financially sound health care system.

Finally, it is a privilege to write this book for you. I look forward to writing future editions with additional timely topics and practical information. If I sell only one book and help one person improve his lifestyle, *Live Longer and Healthier Now!* has served its purpose. I live to make a positive difference in another person's life but I need your help. Physicians can lead their patients to water but we can't make them drink. Take an interest in your health! Compliance with your medications, your physician's advice and the preventive care outlined in this book will help you obtain better health. Life is precious. Consider yourself to be top priority. Take care of yourself first, and then you can tackle the troubles and treasures of your life.

Appendix A

Diabetes Wisdom

Diabetes is a serious disease that has a mortality rate that is the same as cancer. With proper motivation and knowledge, you can change your own future. Diabetes is the seventh-leading cause of death in the USA and affects nearly 16 million people, costing society 100 billion dollars per year. Compliance with your medication, diet, blood monitoring and physician follow-up are essential.

- Type 1, or insulin-dependent, diabetes has a small genetic component and may be caused by a virus or by our own immune system.

- Type 2, or noninsulin-dependent, diabetes has a strong genetic component and is increasing rapidly. The insulin produced by the body doesn't work well and eventually the cells in the pancreas that produce insulin burn out. This disease is affecting an increasing number of adolescents and young adults due to obesity, lack of exercise and perhaps computers and TV. Other rarer causes of diabetes include iron overload, medications such as cortisone, pancreatic cancer, Cushing's syndrome and polycystic ovaries.

- The diagnosis is based on having a fasting blood sugar over 125 or a random sugar over 160. The most sensitive test for diabetes is a sugar testing done 2 hours after a sugary breakfast, such as toast, jelly and orange juice. If it is over 200, you have the disease. The higher the 2-hour postprandial sugar, the greater the risk for heart disease.

- Symptoms of diabetes can include weight loss, increased thirst and increased frequency of urination. Often there are no symptoms, and periodic screening during your physical exam is advised.

- Prevent type 2 diabetes by lifestyle changes. Exercising two and a half hours per week combined with a low-calorie, low-fat diet reduced the new onset of diabetes by 58% in obese sedentary patients. Lifestyle changes worked better than drugs or placebo in the prevention of this disease.

- Seek out a registered dietician to review dietary measures that are recommended by the American Diabetic Association. Avoid simple sugars such as candy or juices as abrupt rises in sugar can occur. Fish, vegetables and fruits are excellent choices.

- Exercise helps to prevent coronary disease and reduces blood pressure. Walking daily for 20 to 30 minutes can reduce heart attacks by 50%. If you are on insulin, take your blood sugar before exercising since physical exertion will reduce the sugar and allow insulin to work better. Drugs that probably reduce the incidence of diabetes include statins like Pravachol, ACE inhibitors like Altace and metformin or Glucophage.

- Self-monitoring is important. Aim for sugars that are 80 to 120 before breakfast and 100 to 140 before bedtime. Also occasionally check your blood sugar 2 hours after a meal. The goal for this sugar measurement is below 140. Blood tests done in the doctor's office are plasma levels as opposed to blood serum levels, which are measured by fingerstick devices. Plasma levels are 10 to 15% higher than blood serum levels. Glucose meters rated highest by *Consumer Reports* include Accu-chek Advantage, One Touch Ultra and Free Style. These meters are accurate and easy to use. Both One Touch and Free Style can be used to sample sugars from the forearm, which is less painful but not quite as accurate as from the fingertips. Don't use the forearm if you are testing the sugar 2 hours after exercising, eating or taking insulin. Laser lancets such as Lasette may be used if you are afraid of needles; however, the pain is the same using a lancet or a needle. Type 2 diabetics may need to test their sugars only once a week before breakfast, depending on the sugar control. Type 1 diabetics will need to test more frequently. Please keep a record of your sugars to show your doctor.

- Hypertension is very common with diabetics and must be aggressively treated, because by so doing one can reduce strokes, end-stage kidney disease and heart attacks. Aim for 130/85 or less as a goal. If you have any protein in the urine, the pressure should be lowered to 125/75 or less. ACE inhibitors such as Altace are indicated to reduce pressure and control protein in the urine. Altace at 10 mg daily can reduce strokes, heart attacks and heart failure as well. ARBs such as Diovan, Avapro and Cozaar can be used if ACE inhibitors are not tolerated. ACE inhibitors commonly cause cough as a side effect. Cozaar is approved for the prevention of end-stage kidney disease and, as with the ACE inhibitors, reduces protein in the urine.

- Vaccinations are very important to prevent the flu and

pneumonia. Obtain the flu vaccine yearly and the pneumonia vaccine every 5 years until age 65. If you are allergic to eggs, do not take these vaccines.

- An eye exam should be performed by an ophthalmologist on a yearly basis. By looking at the vessels in the eye, your doctor can assess damage done to the retina by diabetes (retinopathy) and by high blood pressure.

- The foot examination is very important since diabetics are at increased risk for foot ulcers and amputations. Consider having a podiatrist look at your feet yearly. Inspect your own feet for fungus (white stuff between the toes), cracks, ulcers, drainage, etc. Moisturize your feet especially in the winter to prevent cracking and skin breakdown. Notify your doctor if you see signs of infection as listed above.

- Weight loss can be very useful in controlling diabetes. Aim for a 10% body weight loss by walking and following an ADA diet. If you can maintain a 10% body weight loss at the end of 1 year, you are doing better than most. If you are 100% over your ideal body weight and cannot shed the pounds, consider a gastric bypass or reversible stomach banding through a qualified surgeon.

- Smoking is a deadly habit especially if you have diabetes. Consider the use of Zyban, the nicotine patch, and counseling to help you quit.

- Cholesterol control is also essential to decrease the risk of heart attack and stroke. Aim for a cholesterol under 200, an LDL (bad cholesterol) under 100, an HDL (good cholesterol) over 45 and triglycerides (fats) under 150.

Exercise and diet (peanuts, fruits, vegetables, oatmeal, Benecol, soy, etc.) can help you to obtain these goals. Statin drugs (Zocor, Pravachol, Lipitor, Crestor, LescolXL and Mevacor) are almost essential medications to take if you are diabetic. Zocor and Pravachol have the most evidence with regards to lowering heart attack risk. Monitor liver enzymes and CPK (a muscle test) while on these agents. If you develop new muscle aches, notify your physician. Niacin (Niaspan) can also be helpful to raise HDL and lower triglycerides. Flushing is a common side effect, which can be helped by taking an aspirin one-half hour before taking this medication. Tricor and Gemfibrozil are effective agents at lowering triglycerides and raising HDL but can cause muscle aches or breakdown when combined with a statin drug.

- Aspirin is known to reduce heart attacks by 20% in patients that have multiple risk factors for heart disease. If you are diabetic, consider taking a baby aspirin or regular aspirin daily. Avoid aspirin if you are allergic to it or have stomach ulcers.

- ACE inhibitors are drugs that can help prevent progression of kidney damage induced by hypertension and diabetes. Definitely take these agents if you are spilling protein in the urine or have hypertension. Some experts believe that all diabetics should be on ACE inhibitors even if there is no hypertension or protein in the urine. Your doctor should measure for protein (microalbumin) in your urine at least yearly. Examples of ACE inhibitors include Zestril, Altace, Aceon, Accupril, etc.

- Tight sugar control is important to prevent the complications of diabetes, which include damage to the nerves, eyes and kidneys. The latest goals of treatment include aiming for a fasting sugar of less than 110, an A1C less than 6.5% and a 2-hour postprandial sugar of less than 140. A1C is a blood test that measures the amount of sugar attached to the red cells over a 3-month period of time. This test provides an average of the sugar over the last 3 months, particularly the last month. A low blood count may underestimate your true sugar average. Repeat this test every 3 months. The higher the A1C, the greater the risk of heart attack.

- Hypoglycemia can be a result of trying to maintain a low blood sugar, hence this is an important subject. Symptoms may include nausea, sweating, palpitations, confusion and even coma. A low blood sugar may not afford you enough time to take a piece of candy or a glass of orange juice to counteract it. At least 15 grams of sugar is necessary to counter a low blood sugar. A glucagon emergency kit can be a lifesaver. Glucagon can easily be injected and will raise blood sugar. It is important to instruct a co-worker, friend or family member how to use this kit in case you are not alert enough to use it. All type 1 diabetics should have this kit, and many type 2 diabetics who are at risk for hypoglycemia should have this kit as well.

- Oral agents for diabetes include the sulfonylureas (Amaryl, Glucotrol, glyburide), which stimulate the pancreas to produce insulin, the biguanides (Glucophage), which decrease sugar output from the liver, the TZDs (Avandia and Actos), which lower insulin resistance. Starlix and Prandin stimulate insulin production for a short time and are useful before meals. The highest risk of hypoglycemia results from taking the sulfonylurea drugs. While the risk is still low, hypoglycemia from these drugs especially occurs in the late afternoon. Glucophage shouldn't be used in patients with kidney malfunction, heart failure or liver disease since the risk of lactic acidosis (acid blood) increases. Take this drug with food since nausea and diarrhea are the most common side effects. This agent may result in some weight loss. Actos and Avandia should be used with caution in people with heart failure since some individuals may develop fluid weight gain. These two medications help protect the beta cells in the pancreas that make insulin. Monitor liver tests every 2 months on this drug for the first year and then periodically.

- Insulin is always needed in type 1 diabetics and often needed in type 2 diabetics. Diabetes can be progressive and the oral drugs will eventually not work effectively. The first sugar before breakfast sets the tone for the rest of the day. It is clearly the most important sugar to control. Lantus insulin is excellent at accomplishing this goal. This is a peakless insulin that lasts 24 hours and has demonstrated better sugar control and less hypoglycemia at night than NPH insulin. This insulin is clear, may sting a bit with injection and may not be mixed with other insulins. While this insulin is great to control sugars before meals, a rapid-acting insulin or oral agent should be used to control sugars after eating. Humalog (lispro) or Novalog (insulin Aspart) insulin are rapid-acting insulins that should be given right before eating as opposed to regular insulin, which should be given 30 minutes before a meal. These insulins control sugars as well as regular insulin but result in less hypoglycemia because they don't last as long. Finally, Humalog can be combined with NPH in an insulin pen and injected before breakfast and dinner. The pen should be tipped 10 to 20 times before injecting to avoid the formation of insulin clumps. With any injection make sure that the insulin is filled up to the hub of the needle to avoid injecting air. In type 2 diabetics, Lantus may be combined with Starlix or Amaryl, for example, to maintain sugar control. Eventually rapid-acting insulin spray will be approved for postprandial control. Insulin needles should be disposed properly. Disintegrator Plus is a nifty device that heats the needle and processes it for safe disposal.

- Insulin pumps can be utilized to achieve good control in diabetics. The pumps cost about $5,000 and are often covered by insurance companies and eventually Medicare. A cartridge of 300 units of regular insulin is inserted in the pump, and it is connected subcutaneously in the abdomen via a needle. About half of the insulin is infused slowly over 24 hours, and the rest is given in bolus form just before meals. Eventually these pumps will be able to measure sugar levels as well.

- Glucowatch (wear like a wristwatch) measures sugars every half-hour through the skin. It will not be accurate for immediate readings but may provide an overall idea of your sugar control during the day.

- Stress and depression can accompany diabetes. Be sure to get this treated since diabetes requires a lot of responsibility on your part. If you are unmotivated and can't concentrate well due to depression, it will be harder for you and your physician to control this disease.

- Pancreatic cell transplants into a liver of the diabetic patient provide hope for cure in the future.

- Security in airports continues to heighten. Glucagon kits and insulin bottles with syringes must contain a pharmacy label. Prescriptions or letters from your doctor are not acceptable. Call your airlines before you leave for updated information as these rules are subject to change.

- Wear an alert bracelet or necklace to indicate that you are diabetic. Talk to your pharmacy about obtaining this important item.

- See your physician every 3 months, monitor your sugars, comply with taking your medications and read this appendix again and again.

Appendix B

Body Mass Index (BMI)

The table on the next page has already done the math and metric conversions. To use the table, find your appropriate height (no shoes) in the left-hand column. Move across the row to your approximate weight. The number at the top of the column is the BMI for that height and weight. Seventy percent of the U.S. population is overweight or obese.

BMI (kg/m²)	19	20	21	22	23	24	25	26	27	28	29	30	35	40
Ht. (in.)	Weight (lb.)													
58	91	96	100	105	110	115	119	124	129	134	138	143	167	191
59	94	99	104	109	114	119	124	128	133	138	143	148	173	198
60	97	102	107	112	118	123	128	133	138	143	148	153	179	204
61	100	106	111	116	122	127	132	137	143	148	153	158	185	211
62	104	109	115	120	126	131	136	142	147	153	158	164	191	218
63	107	113	118	124	130	135	141	146	152	158	163	169	197	225
64	110	116	122	128	134	140	145	151	157	163	169	174	204	232
65	114	120	126	132	138	144	150	156	162	168	174	180	210	240
66	118	124	130	136	142	148	155	161	167	173	179	186	216	247
67	121	127	134	140	146	153	159	166	172	178	185	191	223	255
68	125	131	138	144	151	158	164	171	177	184	190	197	230	262
69	128	135	142	149	155	162	169	176	182	189	196	203	236	270
70	132	139	146	153	160	167	174	181	188	195	202	207	243	278
71	136	143	150	157	165	172	179	186	193	200	208	215	250	286
72	140	147	154	162	169	177	184	191	199	206	213	221	258	294
73	144	151	159	166	174	182	189	197	204	212	219	227	265	302
74	148	155	163	171	179	186	194	202	210	218	225	233	272	311
75	152	160	168	176	184	192	200	208	216	224	232	240	279	319
76	156	164	172	180	189	197	205	213	221	230	238	246	287	328

A normal BMI is 19 to 25 (healthy body weight). Overweight is a BMI between 25 and 30. Obesity is a BMI of 30 or more.

Appendix C

Osteoporosis Wisdom

- Osteoporosis is often a silent disease that affects more than 25 million Americans and is manifested by reduced bone density. It results in 1.5 million fractures a year, especially of the spine, hip and wrist (many times the fractures are silent and not apparent to the person).

- Osteoporosis kills more people than breast cancer at age 75. Thirty to forty percent of patients with hip fractures are dead one year later. This costs the USA more than 10 billion dollars a year. This disease can be prevented.

- Risk factors include female sex, white Caucasian, early menopause, blonde hair and blue eyes, smoking and alcohol, steroids, thyroid and other medications, family history, short stature, vitamin D deficiency, malnutrition, thyroid disease, parathyroid disease, rheumatoid arthritis, kidney disease and aging. Most women lose bone mass as a result of menopause and aging. These other conditions should be considered, since some of the factors are modifiable.

- The diagnosis may be established by a bone density measurement. Look at the T-score. This number compares your bone density against that of 35-year-old women. If it is negative 2.5 or more, you have osteoporosis. A score between negative 1 and negative 2.5 represents osteopenia (decreased bone density but not as bad as osteoporosis). Any score higher than negative 1 is normal.

- Accurate measurements of bone density include scans of any of the following bones: hip, spine, finger, forearm and heel. The amount of radiation is about 1/100th of an X ray. Heel ultrasounds may also reflect bone density and architecture.

- Women 25 to 50 should take 1,000 mg of elemental calcium a day with food. If you are over 50, take 1,200 to 1,500 mg a day. Men require about 1,000 mg of calcium a day. A study on 3,270 French women showed that when 1,200 mg of calcium was combined with 800 units of vitamin D, there was a 30% decrease in the risk of hip fractures. One-half cup of sardines or tofu, a cup of milk or yogurt or a glass of calcium-fortified juice each contain 300 mg of calcium. Your diet will contain an additional 200 mg of calcium. Vitamin D deficiency is quite common even with adequate supplementation. This vitamin helps to prevent fractures of bones other than the spine. This vitamin is increased by exposure to the sun. One inexpensive idea would be to take our superb vitamin, the Mega Multiple 85 (www.advancedvitamins.com), which contains 400 units of vitamin D, and add Tums. Each tablet contains calcium carbonate. Calcium and vitamin D will help decrease fractures of both the spine and hip. Other alternatives include Oscal (chewable or oral tablet) or Viactiv (a good-tasting, chewable, chocolate-flavored calcium carbonate). All the above calcium products should be taken in divided doses at meals. Citracal (calcium citrate) is a tablet that is well absorbed when taken between meals. This calcium preparation is better absorbed in the elderly or in people with reduced stomach acid. Medications such as Nexium, Prilosec, Prevacid, Zantac, etc., can reduce stomach acid. Take your pick, but make sure you get adequate calcium and vitamin D! Older folks derive significant benefits from vitamin D including decreased falls and increased muscle strength. This likely results from increased muscle uptake of calcium, which helps the muscle contract.

- Brisk walking and weight-bearing exercises are important. (Try a trainer.)

- Prevent falls by using a night light and eliminating loose rugs and lamp cords. Weight training reduces falls in the elderly. Make sure vision and gait problems are corrected, and avoid medications that cause drowsiness if possible.

- Estrogen therapy reduces hip and spine fractures and works best during the first 5 years after menopause. It reduces overall fracture rate by 25%. It does not help women who already have heart disease. One large trial shows when estrogen is combined with progesterone, an increase in breast cancer, heart disease, stroke and lung clots are seen. Estrogen therapy also may protect against colon cancer and Alzheimer's. It also lowers LDL, or bad cholesterol, and raises HDL, or good cholesterol; however, it raises fats or triglycerides. Finally, epidemiological studies show a trend toward longer life. It is approved for the prevention but not the treatment of osteoporosis. Estrogen definitely helps with menopausal symptoms such as hot flashes, night sweats and vaginal dryness. Due to the benefits and risks of this drug, discuss estrogen replacement therapy with your health care provider.

- Fosamax, at 10 mg per day, increases bone density by 9% in the spine and 6% in the hip after using it for 3 years. It reduces fracture by 50% and prevents height loss. A daily 5-mg dosage should be used if you have osteopenia. This dosage will stabilize bone density. Heartburn is a noted side effect. Take this medication with a full glass of water and at least one-half hour before breakfast or medicine. It is approved for the treatment and prevention of osteoporosis. It is quite effective but inconvenient to take. A once-a-week 70-mg dose is available. Fosamax also works in men.

- Actonel at 5 mg a day or 35 mg once per week can help reduce back fractures by over 60% after one year. It also works at other sites including the hip, forearm and wrist. It must be taken in the same way as Fosamax. There may be less acid reflux (heartburn) with this agent than with Fosamax.

- Didronel (similar to Fosamax) cycled with calcium (400 mg of Didronel for 2 weeks followed by 500 mg of calcium for 11 weeks, and keep repeating) presents a cheaper alternative and increases bone density by 6% in the spine and 2% in the hip. It reduces spine fractures and may help to reduce hip fractures.

- Miacalcin nasal spray is sprayed in alternating nostrils daily and is well tolerated. Rarely sneezing, nausea or flushing occurs. It must be refrigerated until it is opened and used. It is indicated for use beginning 5 years after menopause for the prevention of spinal fractures. Hip-fracture prevention is not proven yet but is being investigated. Its main advantage is convenience of use. It is also approved for the treatment of osteoporosis. Finally, it can reduce the pain associated with osteoporotic fractures.

- Evista (raloxifene), a selective estrogen receptor modulator, increases bone density by 2.5% in the hip and spine. It lowers bad cholesterol (LDL) and CRP but does not raise triglycerides (fats) or HDL (good cholesterol). Compare this with estrogen, which raises triglycerides but also increases the good cholesterol (HDL). Evista causes hot flashes, so it should not be used in women who are having menopausal symptoms. The drug does not stimulate the uterus or breast and may actually prevent breast cancer. By lowering CRP, this medication may actually reduce heart disease. This matter is presently being investigated. Evista may be used along with other medication, for example, Fosamax, for osteoporosis prevention or treatment. It is approved for the treatment and prevention of osteoporosis.

- Forteo is injectable human parathyroid hormone. it increases bone denstiy by 9 to 13% and can reduce fractures in the spine by 65% and at other sites by 55%. Lie down if you experience dizziness or increased heart rate. This drug is injected on a daily basis and should be reserved for use in individuals who are at high risk for osteoporosis. Consider using Forteo if you have had a history of the following: very low bone density, frequent falls, previous fracture on standard medication, intolerance to osteoporosis medication, etc.

Appendix D

Depression and Anxiety Wisdom

- Remember both anxiety and depression are biochemical diseases that are partly determined by our own genes! Scientists can actually show changes that occur in the brain by doing a pet scan. It's not your fault, but don't blame somebody else either. Take care of yourself first and get professional help.

- Common symptoms of depression include feeling down, not experiencing pleasure, difficulty in concentration, agitation, guilt, low energy, insomnia, weight loss, weight gain, suicidal thoughts (common complaint in two-thirds of depressed people) and a plan for suicide (a medical emergency). Multiple physical complaints increase the probability that depression is present. People at higher risk for depression include individuals with a family history of this disease, serious medical ailments, elderly, women, etc. There is nearly a 20% lifetime risk of developing depression. It sounds as though a lot of people have this problem. Elderly Caucasian men have a sixfold risk of committing suicide. Heart attack patients develop depression frequently. Depression also increases the mortality of many chronic diseases. Don't give up hope because there are many successful strategies!

- Common symptoms of anxiety include restlessness, irritability, insomnia, palpitations, breathing problems, stomach distress, etc.

- If you suffer from depression and anxiety, you're in good company. Did you know that Abraham Lincoln had two nervous breakdowns and said that he could turn all the smiles in America to frowns? Winston Churchill and John Lennon suffered from these ailments as well. Obviously, these diseases are not a sign of weakness.

- Spouses, family and friends may become frustrated with depressed and anxious loved ones, but don't expect them to snap out of it. Empathize, be supportive and encourage professional assistance.

- Before any treatment commences, other medical illnesses need to be ruled out. Certain drugs can contribute to depression; these include beta blockers, interferon, oral contraceptives, alcohol and Valium-like agents. Caffeine and pseudoephedrine may aggravate anxiety. Specific illnesses that can cause anxiety or depression include vitamin B12 deficiency (especially if your level is less than 400), thyroid disease, dementia, cancer, sleep disorders, etc. Usually these diseases are not present, but a thorough physical exam and laboratory evaluation should be performed by your health care provider. Women who are postpartum or menopausal may also develop depression.

- Once this is done, you may decide to be treated with medication by your internist/family doctor or psychiatrist. Psychotherapy can be performed by a social worker, psychologist or psychiatrist. The choice should be up to you and your health care adviser. Keep your life simple by avoiding tough decisions and major projects such as moving, quitting smoking, weight loss, etc., during this difficult time.

- How do we treat these ailments? Nondrug treatments include listening to pleasing music, listening to tapes (designed to help reprogram your subconscious, available at your local bookstore), viewing art and exercising regularly. Exercise helps to produce endorphins, which are happy hormones. Some studies show efficacy equivalent to antidepressants. Vince Lombardi, the winning Green Bay Packers coach, once said that exercise is 90% inspiration and 10% perspiration. You may be lacking the motivation if you are anxious or depressed, therefore just try a pleasant walk. Consider being around friends and family members who are helpful to you. Do you need to go to parties? If this activity is pleasant for you, go ahead and participate. The way you think during depression is also important. Avoid the following thoughts: all-or-none thinking (either "I'm perfect or a failure"), overgeneralization ("I'm never understood"; avoid words such as *always* or *never*), negativism ("I'm the cause of all the problems," or "I made a mistake, hence I must be a loser"), etc. Counter any negative thoughts with a positive one. This will be hard to do at first, but will become easier with time. Thoughts such as "I believe in me" or "I am a flexible individual" will help change your internal beliefs. Many of our depressing thoughts come from our underlying belief systems. For example, if your spouse or your boss says that you really messed up a particular task, does that mean you're worthless? If you have this feeling, it is based on a belief that you have somehow developed. Did you base this belief on the words of your boss? This is likely a faulty belief and needs to be changed. One way to change this belief is to constantly say to yourself, "I believe in me" whenever the faulty belief comes to mind. Imagery can work too. Bring up an image of when you accomplished a task that made you feel good inside. Counter the negative with a positive, and you'll feel the difference because your beliefs are changing.

- Light therapy can be helpful if you have seasonal affective disorder. Apparently photo therapy can be effective, especially in the wintertime when there is less sun available. Even glasses that emit light at the right frequency can be purchased. Often they are worn in the morning for 30 to 60 minutes.

- Natural medicines with efficacy in treating depression include SAMe, St. John's wort, and fish oil. Vitamin B complex may have some efficacy and is well tolerated. It may turn your urine a golden yellow, so don't be alarmed!

- SSRIs, or selective serotonin reuptake inhibitors, increase the amount of serotonin in the brain. These agents are nonaddicting and have a 70% chance of working for depression. Examples include Zoloft, Prozac (also generic), Prozac weekly (taken once a week), Celexa, Lexapro, Paxil and Effexor XR. Effexor XR and Paxil are approved for anxiety even without depression. Zoloft and Paxil are approved for posttraumatic stress disorder as well as depression. Prozac (Sarafem) and Zoloft are also approved for premenstrual syndrome. Some 80 to 85% of patients have no side effects on these agents, but some people will develop nausea, diarrhea, sexual dysfunction, etc. These agents take about 2 to 4 weeks to work and should be continued at least a year. Sudden withdrawal of these agents except for Prozac and possibly Celexa can cause symptoms such as dizziness, mood swings, bowel changes, etc. Therefore, slow tapering under your doctor's advice is always wise. Effexor XR, Celexa and Lexapro are the least likely antidepressants to have interactions with other drugs. The S isomer of Celexa, called Lexapro, was released in late 2002 and is similar to Celexa but works more quickly (within 1 to 2 weeks).

- Other antidepressants include Remeron, Serzone and Wellbutrin. All three of these have less effect on sexual dysfunction. Remeron can cause weight gain, which may be helpful in the elderly. Wellbutrin also works for smoking cessation in the form of Zyban. It should not be used for the treatment of anxiety. It can be combined with an SSRl to help with sexual dysfunction, and it can be associated with weight loss.

- Benzodiazepines such as Xanax (alprazolam), Ativan (lorazepam) and Klonopin (clonazepan) can be used for anxiety. These agents are useful for depression initially, if you can't sleep or feel agitated. These drugs are potentially addicting. Nonaddicting drugs for anxiety include BuSpar and Kava Kava, an over-the-counter herb. This herb may be effective at 60 mg of kavalactones (the active ingredient) 3 times daily; however, it can cause liver damage.

- Anxiety and depression commonly relapse. If a person has 2 separate episodes of depression, the chances of having a third one are greater than 90%. If you fall into this category, a prolonged course (years) of antidepressants is usually indicated.

- Medicines that possibly can help to make an antidepressant work better include lithium, thyroid, Zyprexa, BuSpar and other classes of antidepressants.

- If antidepressants cause you to be reckless, have racing thoughts and feel invulnerable, you may be experiencing a manic episode (bipolar disease) and a psychiatrist may need to manage this ailment.

- Be patient with the above medications. Many therapeutic trials may need to be given before the right drug is found. More than 90% of depressed or anxious patients can be helped. Never discontinue a medication or start an herb without input from your doctor. Please consult with your physician regarding this appendix. Finally, remember that anxiety and depression are chemical, so don't be so hard on yourself. Flexible thinking is very important. Yesterday is history, tomorrow's a mystery and today is a gift. In other words, for your own sake forgive the past, don't worry about the future and live each precious day peacefully.

Appendix E

Sleep Wisdom

Common Symptoms of Sleep Disorders

- When did the problem begin (acute or chronic)? Acute problems are often due to stress and are usually short lived.

- Are you down, or not interested in fun activities? Depression commonly wakes you up in the middle of the night and is treated with psychotherapy and antidepressants.

- Do you get attacks of anxiety out of the blue, with symptoms such as choking, sweating, palpitations, warm flushes or feelings of dying? Panic disorder is often treated with low doses of antidepressants such as Paxil or Zoloft.

- Do you have racing thoughts? Do you have increased sex or uncontrollable buying sprees? Do you have little or no need for sleep (manic)?

- Are you nervous and feel irritable and on edge (anxiety)?

- Are there medical conditions that might disrupt sleep? These conditions may be menopause, heartburn, ulcer, enlarged prostate, urination problems, heart failure, emphysema, allergic disorders, seizure, pain, arthritis, fibromyalgia, thyroid disease.

- Are you on prescription drugs that can affect sleep? Such drugs include Ritalin, theophylline, decongestants, antidepressants, diet medication, quinidine, albuterol, alcohol, nicotine, caffeine, steroids, levodopa, beta blockers, etc.

- Is the bedroom too hot, cold or noisy (environmental issues)?

- Are you a shift worker? Do you nap in the daytime? Has there been jet lag?

- Do you have a creepy, crawly feeling in your legs or do you jerk your legs frequently (restless legs syndrome or myoclonic jerks)?

- Do you snore loudly or choke and gasp for breath? Do you feel sleepy or fatigued in the daytime? Do you have high blood pressure, memory problems or erection difficulty (possible sleep apnea)?

- What are the bedtimes and the rising times on weekends and weekdays? (This may relate to poor sleep hygiene.)

- Do you go to bed early and wake up early, or do you go to bed late and wake up late? (These may be advanced sleep disorder or delayed sleep disorder, which are circadian rhythm disorders.)

- Do you fall asleep quickly during the day and experience sleep paralysis on awakening? Do you get weak in the knees or hips in response to strong emotion (narcolepsy)?

- Do you have purposeful behavior during dream sleep? In other words, do you act out your dreams (REM behavior disorder)?

- Do you go to bed with the TV on or feel stressed when you get in bed (conditioned insomnia or psychophysiologic insomnia)?

Answers to Some of the Common Sleep Disorders

- Sleep apnea can be treated by losing weight, avoiding sedatives (Sonata and Ambien are all right), treating hypothyroidism, using CPAP (a pressurized mask that is very effective but noncompliance is common), doing laser UPP (much of the soft palate is removed via a laser; 50% effective in highly selective patients) or by utilizing dental appliances (may decrease apneas by 50% and better compliance than CPAP).

- Restless legs and nocturnal myoclonus (periodic leg movements) can also be treated. Iron deficiency and kidney failure are two common causes of restless legs syndrome. Exercise and hot baths before bedtime may help. Medicines for both these conditions include Sinemet, Mirapex, Permax, Klonopin, Neurontin and Vicodin.

- Circadian rhythm disorders can be effectively treated by using sunlight (light therapy). Advance-phase disorders can be treated with sunlight in the evening so the person will go to bed later. Delayed-sleep disorder can be treated with sunlight in the morning so awakening time will be earlier. One may also buy a portable unit (2,500-lux illuminator).

- Narcolepsy can be treated with stimulants such as Dexedrine or Provigil.

- Psychiatric problems are important to treat. Help depression with psychotherapy and medicine such as Effexor XR (has been used effectively for the most resistant depressions and increases 3 hormones in the brain to effect a chemical change). Panic can be treated with Paxil at low dosages. Mania and psychosis should be treated by a psychiatrist. Anxiety disorders may respond to any of the following drugs: Klonopin, BuSpar, Paxil, Effexor XR and other medications.

- Medical diseases can interrupt sleep. Treat the underlying cause such as heartburn with Prilosec, Protonix, Aciphex, Nexium or Prevacid. Alzheimer's may be treated with Aricept, Exelon or Reminyl. Other medications and diseases that can disrupt sleep are listed above.

Sleep Treatment: A General Guide
Stimulus Control

- Go to bed only when you are sleepy. Do not use the bed for anything except for sleep or sex. Don't read, watch TV or eat in bed. Also remember to wind down before bedtime, for example, by listening to relaxing music.

- If you don't fall asleep in 15 to 20 minutes, leave the bedroom and return when you are sleepy. Repeat as often as necessary until you fall asleep in 15 to 20 minutes.

- Get up at the same time each day no matter how much time you slept.

- Do not nap during the day or sleep in other locations except your bed.

Sleep Hygiene

- Eliminate use of caffeine even in the morning.

- Do not use alcohol or tobacco products near bedtime.

- Avoid naps.

- Wake up at the same time every day.

- Avoid heavy meals at bedtime; light snacks are all right.

- Regular exercise in the afternoon may deepen sleep, but do not exercise within 3 to 4 hours of bedtime.

- Move the alarm clock so you cannot see it, and shut the TV off.

Sleep Restriction

- This technique involves limiting the amount of time in bed. If you lie in bed for 6 hours and only sleep for 4 hours, the next night restrict your time in bed to only 4 hours. Sleep debt accumulates and you get sleepier. Once 85% of time in bed is spent sleeping, the allowable time in bed is slowly increased.

Medicines Used to Treat Sleep Disorders

- Zaleplon (Sonata)–quick onset, half-life equals 1 hour, no effect on sleep architecture, no rebound insomnia, no withdrawal syndrome, minimal coordination impairment and no memory impairment at peak levels, delayed onset with food, total sleep time increased, side effects no greater than placebo, dosage is 5 mg at bedtime (elderly), usually 10 mg at bedtime if younger, no residual next-day effects, minimal addiction.

- Zolpidem (Ambien)–quick onset, half-life equals 2.5 hours, no effect on sleep architecture, rebound insomnia noted on first night, moderate coordination and memory impairment, total sleep time increased, residual next-day effects noted, side effects similar to placebo, same dose as Sonata, minimal addiction.

- Trazodone (Desyrel)–intermediate onset (60 to 120 minutes), may cause persistent erection (1 in 6,000 men) and residual drowsiness, no addiction, 50 to 300 mg may be helpful.

- Diphenhydramine (Benadryl)–intermediate onset, peak levels at 7 hours, residual impairment, disrupts sleep architecture, not good for elderly (confusion and urine retention), found in Tylenol PM, 25 to 50 mg of this drug can help with sleep.

- Melatonin–intermediate onset, may help shift workers and jet lag, may disrupt sleep and cause irritability, daytime drowsiness, depression, and decreased ovulation,1 to 3 mg at bedtime is the usual dose.

Appendix F

Green Tea Capsules

1-866-775-7628 www.DrLipkis.com

- Green tea contains polyphenols, which are powerful antioxidants. A specific polyphenol called EGCG (a catechin) is 20 to 200 times more powerful than vitamin E in its ability to neutralize free radicals. It also neutralizes mutagenic nitrosamines and harmful toxins.

- A 1999 Harvard study showed that drinking a cup of green tea or black tea a day (brewed and without milk) reduced heart attacks by 44%. Green tea probably thins the blood a bit, and thus reduces heart attacks. Consuming 10 cups a day increased HDL (good cholesterol) and decreased LDL (bad cholesterol).

- Epidemiological studies show that rates of breast, colon, skin, pancreatic, esophageal and stomach cancer are less in green tea consumers. Many cups should be consumed. Interestingly, the Japanese have the highest smoking rates but the lowest incidence of lung cancer. Another Japanese study concludes that women with breast cancer who drink 5 cups of green tea daily reduced their likelihood of relapse by 50%. Green tea inhibits blood vessel growth and collagenases, which tumors need to grow and spread.

- Green tea extract may be useful for weight loss. A small study in men demonstrates that supplementation increases 24-hour energy expenditure without any change in heart rate or blood pressure. It seems to be thermogenic and helps to break down fat. Animal studies show decreased fat absorption in the gut.

- Green tea may also help to lower blood sugar by reducing the activity of amylase, which breaks down starches into sugars. It also slows down sugar absorption in the gut. Human trials are ongoing.

- There is a low incidence of rheumatoid arthritis in China, Japan and India where much green tea is consumed. A study in mice showed reduced severity of rheumatoid arthritis. Additionally, green tea helped to prevent this disease. This tea also increases bone density.

- Strokes were reduced by 50% in Japanese women over 40 who drank 5 or more cups of green tea per day. A smaller Dutch study performed in men showed a 70% reduction in strokes with the consumption of black tea (similar to green tea).

- Green tea can kill the flu virus and even demonstrates some activity against the HIV virus. It can also inhibit the growth of oral bacteria including periodontal and decay-causing bacteria.

- All green teas are not alike. It is easy to be deceived with the polyphenol content, hence leave the pickings to me!

- Our inexpensive green tea preparation provides the equivalent of 4 to 5 cups of green tea in each capsule.

Take 2 to 3 capsules daily. You have our money-back guarantee! Order by calling 1-866-775-7628 or on the Web at www.DrLipkis.com. Click on the button that says "Advanced Vitamins." Finally, enter "green tea" in the search box. I know you will be delighted with this product!

Appendix G

Q-Gel (Coenzyme Q-10)

1-866-775-7628 www.DrLipkis.com

- Scientific studies prove that Q-Gel produces higher levels of coenzyme Q-10 in the blood than many other equivalent brands of this outstanding natural vitamin.

- This powerful antioxidant helps prevent the bad cholesterol (LDL) from sticking to our arteries.

- Studies demonstrate that Q-Gel improves congestive heart failure (the number one reason for hospitalization), reduces angina, palpitations and blood pressure.

- Boosts immunity by increasing antibody production.

- Reduces blood sugar readings.

- Q-Gel increases cellular energy and can result in a modest weight loss (fat burning).

- Human studies show healing of gums (improvement of periodontal disease).

- Women with breast cancer and breast lumps have low levels of coenzyme Q-10. Supplementation with Q-Gel is worth doing.

- Lifespan extension has been documented in mammals given coenzyme Q-10 (60% increase in survival).

- Q-Gel helps to increase energy production in the brain, and scientific papers indicate that it may be useful in the prevention and treatment of Alzheimer's, Parkinson's, stroke and Lou Gehrig's disease.

- Q-Gel has a great safety profile.

- Take 1 Q-Gel daily (with or without food) for prevention.

- Take 2 Q-Gel per day if you have heart disease, neurologic problems, diabetes or obesity (30% above ideal body weight). Take 1 to 2 Q-Gel daily for gum disease.

- Buy this exceptional life-enhancing product by calling 1-866-775-7628. Each bottle of Q-Gel provides a 2-month supply guaranteed to your satisfaction or a complete refund will be given. You may also order through our website at www.DrLipkis.com.

References

1   Sinatra, S. *The Coenzyme Q-10 Phenomenon* (1999).
2   "ABC News Tonight with Peter Jennings" (November 1997).
3   Klatz, R., and R. Goldman. *Stopping the Clock* (Keats Publishing Inc., 1996).
4   Blitznakof, E., and G. Hunt. *The Miracle Nutrient: Coenzyme Q-10* (Bantam, 1987).
5   Sahelian, R. *Coenzyme Q-10: Nature's Heart Energizer* (Impact Communications, 1998).

Appendix H

Mega Multiple 85

1-866-775-7628 www.DrLipkis.com

- Superb inexpensive multiple vitamin.

- This vitamin is highly absorbable and comes in an easy-to-swallow capsule form.

- Contains high doses of B vitamins and folic acid, which have been useful for the prevention of coronary disease and stroke. Such vitamins may reduce the incidence of colon cancer by 75%. Additionally, B vitamins may help to prevent Alzheimer's. Finally, these nutrients may help with depression and arthritis.

- Contains magnesium aspartate for energy production.

- Contains no iron. This element may contribute to organ damage, such as heart failure.

- Contains 400 units of vitamin D, which can help prevent osteoporosis. Take this vitamin and you can buy calcium without vitamin D and save.

- The Mega Multiple 85 contains 3 times the vitamin C, 2 times the vitamin A and 30 times the vitamin B as national brands such as Centrum. The cost is similar and this vitamin comes in easy-to-swallow capsules.

- Exercise, eat healthy, obtain regular checkups, take green tea capsules and Q-Gel and add the balance of our inexpensive Mega Multiple.

Bibliography

"Alcoholism." *The Journal of the American Medical Association* 281 (1999): 1318.

"Allergic Rhinitis." *Annals of Allergy, Asthma, and Immunology* 81, pt. 2 (1998): 463.

"Alzheimer's." Paper presented at the meeting of the Society for Neuroscience, Miami Beach, 24 October 1999.

"Alzheimer's Disease." *The Journal of the American Medical Association* 278 (1997): 1363, 1327.

"Alzheimer's Disease." *New England Journal of Medicine* 346 (2002): 476.

Annals of Internal Medicine 131 (1999): 850.

Annals of Internal Medicine 133 (2000): 981.

Annals of Pharmacotherapeutics 35 (2001): 1118.

Archives of Internal Medicine 156 (1996): 2213.

British Journal of Cancer 81 (1999): 1238.

British Medical Journal 317 (1998): 1624.

"Cardiology." *Stroke* 30 (1999): 2502.

"Cholesterol." *New England Journal of Medicine* 341 (1999): 410.

Circulation 98 (1998): 1198.

Circulation 102 (2000): 2296.

Clinical Drug Investigations 17 (1999): 211.

Davis, Lisa. "Holy Cow!" *Reader's Digest* (July 2002): 107–16.

"Dietary Supplements." *Journal of the National Cancer Institute* 90 (1998): 414.

"Dietary Supplements." *Prescriber's Letter* (July 1998; 11

August 2002).

"Does Exercise Encourage a Return to Normal Activities in Low Back Pain Patients?" *Archives of Internal Medicine* 161 (23 April 2001): 1081-88.

European Journal of Clinical Research 9 (1997): 261.

Forum Immunology 8 (1992): 2.

Golden, William E., M.D. "Chronic Fatigue Syndrome." *Internal Medicine News* (1 September 2002): 13.

Graat, Judith, M.S., Evert Schouten, M.D., Ph.D., and Frans Kok, Ph.D. "Effect of Daily Vitamin E and Multivitamin-Mineral Supplementation on Acute Respiratory Tract Infections in Elderly Persons." *The Journal of the American Medical Association* (August 2002): 715–16.

"Herbal Supplements." *Archives of Family Medicine* 7 (1998): 541.

"Infectious Diseases." *Journal of Family Practice* 49 (2000): 907.

"Introduction." *American Family Physician* 62 (2000): 1575, 1587.

Journal of the American Academy of Nurse Practitioners 12 (2000): 311.

The Journal of the American Medical Association 268 (1992): 3462.

The Journal of the American Medical Association 275 (1996): 1389.

The Journal of the American Medical Association 276 (1996): 1957.

The Journal of the American Medical Association 277 (1997): 887.

The Journal of the American Medical Association 281 (1999): 1112.

The Journal of the American Medical Association 282 (1999): 1233.

Journal of Clinical Oncology 20 (2002): 1449.

Journal of Family Practice 47 (1998): 118.

Journal of the National Cancer Institute 91 (1999): 317.

Journal of Rheumatology 23 (1996): 5.

Kivipeito, Miia, M.D. "Apolipoprotein E e4 Allele, Elevated Midlife Total Cholesterol Level, and High Midlife Systolic Blood Pressure Are Independent Risk Factors for Late-Life Alzheimer Disease." *Annals of Internal Medicine* (6 August 2002): 149.

Lancet 347 (1996): 781.

Lancet 348 (1996): 429.

Lancet 349 (1997): 1710, 1715.

Leikin, Jerrold, M.D. *Poisoning and Toxicology Handbook* (2002).

"Massage for Chronic Back Pain? Better Than a Poke in the Skin with a Sharp Stick?" *British Medical Journal* 319 (31 July 1999): 279-83.

The Medical Letter on Drugs and Therapeutics 40 (1999): 117.

Morbidity and Mortality Weekly Report 48, RR-6 (1999): 1-6.

Neuroepidemiology 17 (1998): 14.

Neurology 43 (1993): 1609.

Neurology 54 (2000): 240.

"Neurology/Psychiatry." *Journal of the American Geriatric Society* 44 (1996): 1307.

"Neurology/Psychiatry." *Prescriber's Letter* (September 2002).

"New Bethesda Terminology and Management Guidelines for Pap Smear Findings." *The Journal of the American Medical Association* 287 (24 April 2002): 2114–19.

New England Journal of Medicine 340 (1999): 1482.

New England Journal of Medicine 342 (2000): 1484.

"Oncology." *Cancer Research* 62 (2002): 2474.

"Oncology." *Lancet* 357 (2001): 1764.

Onion, Daniel. *Blackwell's Primary Care Essentials* (2003).

"Ophthalmology." *Prescriber's Letter* (26 August 2002).

Owsley, Cynthia MSPH, Ph.D., Gerald McGown, Jr., MS, Ph.D., Michael Sloane, Ph.D., Jennifer Wells, LBSW,

CDRS, Beth T. Stalvey, MPH, Ph.D., and Scott Gavthreavx, M.D. "Impact of Cataract Surgery on Motor Vehicle Crash Involvement by Older Adults." *The Journal of the American Medical Association* (21 August 2002): 841.

"Parkinson's Disease." *Neurology,* suppl. 5 (2001): 56.

Parmet, Sharon, MS. "Carbon Monoxide Poisoning." *The Journal of the American Medical Association* (28 August 2002): 1036.

"Pediatrics." *Pediatrics* 105 (2000): 84, 136.

Peterson, Lyle, M.D., M.P.H., and Anthony A. Marfin, M.D., M.P.H. "West Nile Virus: A Primer for the Clinician." *Annals of Internal Medicine* (6 August 2002): 173.

"Prostate Cancer." *Journal of the National Cancer Institute* 90 (1998): 440, 1184, 1219.

"Prostate Cancer: Early Detection." *New Horizons* (September 2001): 1–24.

Psychopharmacology Bulletin 31 (1995): 147.

"Respiratory/Allergy." *New England Journal of Medicine* 343 (2000): 332.

"Rheumatoid Arthritis." *Arthritis and Rheumatology* 46 (2002): 328.

Solomon, Paul, Ph.D., Felicity Adams, B.A., Amanda Silver, B.A., Jill Zimmer, B.A., and Richard DeVeaux, Ph.D. "Ginkgo for Memory Enhancement: A Randomized Controlled Trial." *The Journal of the American Medical Association* (21 August 2002): 835.

"Statins." Paper presented at American Heart Association Scientific Sessions 2001, Anaheim, 30 November 2001.

"Statins." *Prescriber's Letter* (December 2001; 16 September 2002).

Straus, Sharon, M.D., Sumit Majumdar, M.D., and Finlay McAllister, M.D. "New Evidence for Stroke Prevention." *The Journal of the American Medical Association* (18 September 2002): 1388–94.

Stroke 30 (1999): 1772.

www.stroke.org.

Zeitschreift Phytother 13 (1992): 7.

Index

A

Accidents, preventing
    and alcohol, 65-66
    in automobile, 65-66
    in boating, 66
    and lightning, 69-70
    and Medic Alert
        devices, 88
    and poison alert, 88-89
    and smoke detectors, 70
    in sports, 66
ACE inhibitor, 24
    and coronary artery
        disease, 77
    and diabetes, 148, 150
    and heart failure, 82
    and hypertension, 31
    and stroke prevention, 84
Addiction
    alcohol, 13-14
    smoking, 50-52
AIDS virus, 29
Alcoholics Anonymous, 14

Alcoholism, 13-14
    drug treatment for, 14

Allergies, 14-15
    and asthma, 18-19
    drug treatment for, 15
Alpha blockers, 32, 92-93
Alzheimer's, 15-17
    prevention of, 16, 94, 142
    treatment of, 17
Anesthesia, and surgical
    issues, 53
Antibiotics
    and common cold, 22
    and sinusitis, 48-49
Antidepressants, 163-167
    and Alzheimer's, 17
    and fibromyalgia, 27
    and gambling, 28
Antihistamines, 15
Anti-inflammatory agents
    and fibromyalgia, 27

Protective devices, and
accidents, 65-66
PSA test, for prostate cancer, 63
Pulmonary embolus, 46-47

R
Religion, and quality of life,
89
Rheumatoid arthritis, 47-48

S
Saw palmetto, 138-139
Seatbelts, and accident
prevention, 65-66
Self-exams, 56, 125
Sex
and health, 125
and immunity, 23
Sexual dysfunction
in men, 93-94
in women, 97-98
Sexually transmitted disease
(STD), 102-104, 125
chlamydia, 102-103
hepatitis C, 28
herpes, 103
HIV, 29-30
HPV, 102
Sigmoidoscopy, 58
Sinusitis, 48-49
and asthma, 18
and headaches, 35
Skin
cancer, and early
detection, 63-64, 125

Derma Q-Gel cream,
133-134
and sunburn, 63-64
Sleep disorders, 126-127
apnea, 65, 83
medications for, 173
symptoms of, 168-170
treatment of, 170-172
Smallpox, 49-50
Smoke detectors, 70
and carbon monoxide,
68-69
Smoking, 23
and bladder cancer, 55
and cessation, 50-52
and erectile dysfunction,
93
and diabetes, 149
and lung cancer, 60-61
and macular
degeneration, 33
and strokes, 85
Soy products, 97, 139
St. John's wort, 139-140
Statins, 25, 33, 73-74, 77, 79
Street drugs, 70-71
Stress
and back pain, 19
and diabetes, 153
and hypertension, 31
and smoking, 50
Stroke
and heart disease, 84-86
and hypertension, 30
and obesity, 35
prevention of, 84-86

Quick Order Form

Fax Orders: 847-729-8852. Please send this form.

Telephone Orders: Call 866-775-7628 toll free. Have your credit card ready.

Email Orders: www.DrLipkis.com

Postal Orders: Advanced Publishing
                       Evan L. Lipkis MD.
                       2150 Pfingsten Rd. Suite 2200
                       Glenview, Illinois 60025

Please send the book, Live Longer and Healthier Now! to:

Name:_____

Address:_____

City:_____ State:_____ Zip:_____

Telephone:_____

Email address:_____

Price $19.95 plus $4 for shipping and handling. Total cost is $23.95

Payment method:
____check   ____credit card
    ____Visa   ____MasterCard   ____Discover